SOAP MAKING FOR BEGINNERS

How to Make an All-natural Mild and Carefully Crafted Handmade Soap

(Guide to Produce Diy Hand Sanitizer for Personal Hygiene)

Edward Pennin

Published by Oliver Leish

Edward Pennington

All Rights Reserved

Soap Making for Beginners: How to Make an All-natural Mild and Carefully Crafted Handmade Soap (Guide to Produce Diy Hand Sanitizer for Personal Hygiene)

ISBN 978-1-77485-088-6

Legal & Disclaimer

The information contained in this book is not designed to replace or take the place of any form of medicine or professional medical advice. The information in this book has been provided for educational and entertainment purposes only.

The information contained in this book has been compiled from sources deemed reliable, and it is accurate to the best of the Author's knowledge; however, the Author cannot guarantee its accuracy and validity and cannot be held liable for any errors or omissions. Changes are periodically made to this book. You must consult your doctor or get professional medical advice before using any of the suggested remedies, techniques, or information in this book.

Upon using the information contained in this book, you agree to hold harmless the Author from and against any damages, costs, and expenses, including any legal fees potentially resulting from the application of any of the information provided by this guide. This disclaimer applies to any damages or injury caused by the use and application, whether directly or indirectly, of any advice or information presented, whether for breach of contract, tort, negligence, personal injury, criminal intent, or under any other cause of action.

You agree to accept all risks of using the information presented inside this book. You need to consult a professional medical practitioner in order to ensure you are both able and healthy enough to participate in this program.

Table of Contents

INTRODUCTION 1

CHAPTER 1: WHAT ARE THE COSTS INVOLVED IN OPENING A SOAP MAKING BUSINESS? 2

CHAPTER 2: THE DIFFERENT TYPES OF SOAP MAKING 13

CHAPTER 3: SOAP MAKING PROCESSES 26

CHAPTER 4: DIY SOAP 101 46

CHAPTER 5: COMMERCIAL SOAP 56

CHAPTER 6: WHAT GOES INTO SOAP? 84

CHAPTER 7: BEST HOMEMADE SOAP RECIPES 105

CHAPTER 8: EQUIPMENT 115

CHAPTER 9: USING SOAP BASE 127

CHAPTER 10: CHOOSE YOUR POISON 134

CHAPTER 11: SOAP RECIPES YOU CAN MAKE AT HOME. 141

CHAPTER 12: IT'S THYME: HERBAL SOAP MAKING FROM SCRATCH 187

CHAPTER 13: SOAP RECIPES 197

VEGGIES SUDS 1 197

Veggie Suds With Coconut 198

Chocolate Almond Soap... 199

Luxury Castile Bar Soap.. 201

CONCLUSION.. **203**

Introduction

The soap business is a very lucrative business that cannot run out of sales, so in this book, we will teach you how to identify the kinds of soap that work for different people. This book will also teach you how to make these soaps from the comfort of your home and make money from it. Ranging from soaps for the elderly, kids, men, young adults, and for different skin-related issues, this book gives you step by step process of making these soaps from start to finish. In this book, we will list the basic tools needed for starting your soap business and how to promote the business.

Chapter 1: What Are The Costs Involved In Opening A Soap Making Business?

If you have a kitchen or workspace and a few basic kitchenwares, you've got a good start. Soapmaking isn't an expensive business to get into, but there are some basic investments you'll need to make.

• Ingredients -- $200 or more. Soaps are made from lye and fats or oils. That's the starting point, but your unique recipe is what will make you stand out. You could use coconut oil, olive oil, almond oil and a whole host of fragrance oils, extracts and natural additives for superior feel, fragrance and lather qualities. You might start with only one or two basic recipes to contain materials costs and simplify production when you start out.

• Soapmaking equipment -- $300 or more. The type of soapmaking you undertake will determine your equipment needs. There are four basic types of production -- hot process, cold process, rebatching and melt and pour -- and each process requires different equipment. But whichever way you go, you'll also probably need soap molds and packaging and shipping materials. You'll find numerous online vendor sources for your basic ingredients, additives, tools and accessories, including this site.

• Marketing tools -- $750 or more. A professional-looking website with attractive product photos is very important to your business. Your web customers can't feel or smell your products, so they must be able to perceive the high quality in terms of what they see online. That means it's worth the investment of a graphic designer and web developer who can help you get the most out of your logo and digital presence. Your graphic imagery will be carried through in your packaging and labels to express your passion and commitment to product excellence.

• Professional services -- $200 or more. Does your state and community allow you to operate this type of business from your home? Hold a brief meeting with a lawyer before you hang out your shingle.

• Professional association -- $100 annual membership in the Handcrafted Soap & Cosmetics Guild (HSCG). This organization can provide training, support, and valuable networking opportunities for small-quantity soapmakers.

• General liability and product liability insurance -- $265-$375 a year. You'll also find this through the HSCG.

What are the ongoing expenses for a soap making business?

Your largest ongoing expenses will be the consumable product ingredients you'll need for ongoing production. If you've priced your offering wisely, your expanding variable costs will be more than offset by an increase in sales.

Who is the target market?

Most of the market for handmade soaps consists of women, but some handmade soap companies have also found success marketing male-oriented soap scents. You might seek customers who appreciate the quality and luxury of your product, or those who only buy organic or vegan products. Your customers will notice the difference in quality between your soaps and those available on a common store shelf.

How much can you charge customers?

Your products might retail for five- or six-dollars a bar. This is more than your customers will pay for mass-produced supermarket soaps, but the perceived value of your production is high. Also, you can arrive at other price points by discounting for multiple purchases, selling multiple-bar packages, and expanding your product line. Check the websites of nearby competitors to see what they're charging and decide how that will affect your pricing. Will you charge more to connote a more premium product line or charge less and make up for less per-unit profit margin with more volume?

How much profit can a soap making business make?

There are a few famous soapmakers who started much like you. Consider, for instance, Burt's Bees. Others in your business keep it part-time, and somewhere between a crafts hobby and a modestly profitable business. As with a lot of home-based businesses, you can go as far as your commitment, creativity, promotional savviness, and hard work take you.

How can you make your business more profitable?

Many soapmakers expand their menu offering to include other kinds of soaps (goat's milk soap is one exotic example) or complementary products. Candlemaking is a natural extension, especially for soapmakers already using a hot process. Others get into home fragrances, lip balms, hair care products, and even pet products. To consider expanding your own product mix, focus on what else would appeal to your customer base. Many businesses seek to raise their overall profits by driving down the cost to produce the goods. Issuing larger batches at a time is a cost-effective way to maximize your profits.

Form A Legal Entity

Establishing a legal business entity such as an LLC prevents you from being personally liable if your soap making business is sued. There are many business structures to choose from including: Corporations, LLC's, and DBA's. You should also consider using a registered agent service to help protect your privacy and stay compliant.

Register For Taxes

You will need to register for a variety of state and federal taxes before you can open for business. In order to register for taxes you will need to apply for an EIN. It's really easy and free!

Open A Business Bank Account & Credit Card

Using dedicated business banking and credit accounts is essential for personal asset protection. When your personal and business accounts are mixed, your personal assets (your home, car, and other valuables) are at risk in the event your business is sued. In business law, this is referred to as piercing your corporate veil.

Open a business bank account

• This separates your personal assets from your company's assets, which is necessary for personal asset protection.

• It also makes accounting and tax filing easier.

Get a business credit card

• This helps you separate personal and business expenses by putting your business' expenses all in one place.

• It also builds your company's credit history, which can be useful to raise money and investment later on.

Set Up Business Accounting

Recording your various expenses and sources of income is critical to understanding the financial performance of your business. Keeping accurate and detailed accounts also greatly simplifies your annual tax filing.

Obtain Necessary Permits And Licenses

Failure to acquire necessary permits and licenses can result in hefty fines, or even cause your business to be shut down.

State & Local Business Licensing Requirements

Certain state permits and licenses may be needed to operate a handmade soap business. In addition, many states have various rules regulating the production of cosmetics and other body care items.

Get Business Insurance

Insurance is highly recommended for all business owners. If you hire employees, workers compensation insurance may be a legal requirement in your state.

Define Your Brand

Your brand is what your company stands for, as well as how your business is perceived by the public. A strong brand will help your business stand out from competitors.

How to promote & market a soap making business

Look for points of differentiation. For instance, consider making a bar of soap that's larger than usual or formulated to last longer. Perhaps you could sell a six-pack of smaller-size sampler soaps so your customer can affordably try your entire product line and pick favorites. Discover an infrequently used fragrance or additive for texture that makes your soaps unique. Once you've found an idea that works, promote it in your website and on social media. Also, if you're exhibiting your soaps at shows, bring some unwrapped examples of your complete product line so customers can hold them, see what they actually look like, feel their textures, and enjoy the varied scents.

Chapter 2: The Different Types Of Soap Making

There are many different ways to make soap but there are two main processes that people use to create it. There is the cold method (or cold process) and the hot method (or hot process).

All of them work to mix together the fat and the alkali but they vary in how they get the water to evaporate and leave you with just the salt at the end.

The cold process method

The cold method is relatively simple but requires more precision than the hot method.

First you pick a fat and look up the saponification value of it – this is the amount of alkali you need to begin treating it to create soap. Different types of fats need more or less lye to make sure the process results in a neat finished product.

Too much lye and there will be some lye that doesn't react properly. This can make a crumbly soap and raise the pH level so high that it makes it irritating for skin.

If you've ever found soap to be itchy it means the pH was too high for your skin (some people have more tolerance to variations in skin pH). Making your own soap gives you better control over this.

If you put in too much fat and not enough lye, then the soap will be greasy or may not even set properly. Usually people put in a little more fat than they technically need as the potency of the alkali cannot be guaranteed and slightly greasy soap is better than soap that burns your skin.

Cold method soap is no place for a pinch of lye here and there.

The fat and lye need to be in liquid form for them to mix properly. This means you need to melt a solid fat or use liquid oil. You dissolve lye in water and then mix them together and stir until they are fully 'emulsified' and the mixture becomes slightly thick.

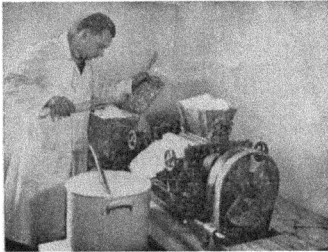

Although called the 'cold method' you will need to warm up the water you use. The 'cold' simply refers to the fact that you don't heat up the soap mixture.

At this point people typically put in their scents and dyes though you can do so earlier if you really know what you are doing. You then put this mixture into some kind of mould and leave them in a warm place for a day or two (usually covered up with a blanket or towel).

Once the soap is firm and can be properly removed from a mould you are then free to start using it. Many people will leave the soap to be cured for a week or two so you are certain all excess lye and water is gone.

For most home soap makers, the cold method is more preferable to the hot one. It's simple, inexpensive, and if you use a good mould and get the measurements right you'll have excellent quality soap. This method also leaves in glycerin which many people find desirable.

The big downside is that if you mess up the mixture you could make soap that is potentially harmful which is much harder to do with the hot method. However, this isn't a concern on a small scale as it's very simple to make sure the mixture is right.

On an industrial scale this process is not only more time consuming, but you could potentially make thousands of soaps that could damage skin.

The hot process method

With the hot method of soap making you are putting the saponification process on fast forward so you can be scrubbing up with your soap much quicker.

As with the cold method you mix together your fat and your lye and then you heat the mixture in a pot up to 90 degrees Celsius. After a while the mixture will turn a thicker gel form and saponification will have taken place.

This gel stage happens with the cold method but it does so while it's hanging around in your warm place for two days. Once you've got it to a gel you add in your smelly stuff and dyes, then you put it in a mould and wait until it cools down before cutting and leaving to dry.

When you make soap like this you don't have to worry so much about the mixtures because the heating makes sure saponification happens and it will definitely enter the gel phase at some point.

The heating phase also allows you to be sure that any additives you put in (scents and dyes) won't do weird things to the soap forming process (for example allowing some of them to not react).

Some oils are also neutered when you place them in the cold method mixture as they have to go through the sopanification process as well. In the hot method the process is essentially complete and you're just adding the ingredients before it sets.

On a final note you will need to use the hot method if you want to make a liquid handsoap and especially if you want it to be colorless. It's also far easier to remove glycerin at this stage.

The melt and pour method

If you want to make soap, there is a third way to do it known as the melt and pour method where you buy some pre-made soap mixture and then melt it and put your own flavors and concoctions in it.

Since it has already technically been made you don't need to worry about using either a hot or cold process to make it. You simply melt down the mixture and then put it in a mould to set.

You can buy a 1kg mixture for under $10 and you are free to experiment and play with it. There are lots of reasons to favor the melt and pour method. Firstly, it's not really more expensive if you are planning on only making a little soap.

Secondly, you don't need to handle lye or bother with safety equipment and you don't need several containers to handle all of your lye and soap making byproducts. You just need a jug and a mould.

If you've never made soap before it might be a good idea to try out a melt and pour first to get an idea of what you can do with it. If you are only really interested in making novelty soaps in weird shapes or with funky colors it might be the case that pour and melt will fit all your needs.

So why wouldn't you use melt and pour? Firstly, it doesn't make particularly great soap. It's perfectly fit for purpose but it won't last as long and may be a little squishier than you want.

Secondly it's not especially cheap. Melt and pour isn't expensive but generally you are paying at least 5 times the price for a similar product you could make using another method.

If you compare say buying coconut oil at a supermarket with the price of buying a pour and melt coconut milk soap base, then the base seems excellent value – but if you look a little further out you can buy coconut oil very cheaply in bulk.

Lastly, and most importantly, you don't have the same choice of fats when you get a pre-made soap mix like this. You are limited to the soap bases on sale and mixing together combinations of fats isn't possible.

If you're serious about making good soap, then melt and pour just won't cut it.

Which process should I choose?

Picking the right process or method for you will depend a lot on your apparatus and what you want to do with your soap.

If you want to make lots of soap relatively quickly then the hot process is clearly the best option. Not only can you have large batches of soap ready in just a few days but you don't have to worry as much about ensuring you have the perfect combination of chemicals.

It's also the best option for liquid soaps, soaps using more reactive dyes and scents, soaps without as much glycerin, and transparent soaps.

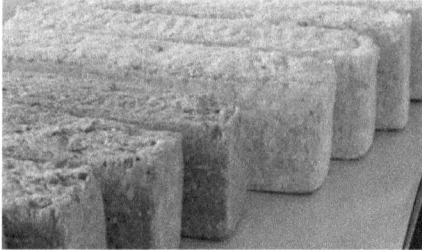

For most beginners, however, the cold process will be preferable – especially if you are only making a smaller quantity of soap. Less apparatus is required and you won't have a lye mixture bubbling over your stove for several hours.

Preparing the soaps for moulds is relatively quick with the cold process and there's no danger of making it too hot and evaporating any oils you put in.

It's the best option if you want opaque solid soaps (especially lighter colored soaps) and you have more flexibility in mixing together different soaps and making patterns.

This can be harder to do with hot gels (which aren't as easy to swirl and spread) and you would need to time things so you have the different gels ready at the right time. So for people looking to make some really wild designs it is easiest to do with the cold process soap.

In addition, some argue that gelled soap isn't as smooth or buttery and you can avoid that with the cold process.

Ultimately both methods are useful and if you are very serious about making soap you will likely experiment with both at some point. You might want to start with the cold process to see if it works, but if you are looking to make a specific type of soap you can easily start with the hot process.

Soap ingredients and apparatus

So you've chosen a process for making your soap so now the question is what do you put in your soap and what do you put those ingredients in to make the soap?

You might have a dream of making a fantastic lemon and mint mojito style soap – and while garden mint and lemon oil will be good enough there are other questions you need to ask before you can begin.

Do you want your soap to lather a lot? Do you want big and fluffy bubbles or none at all? Do you want hard soap, brittle soap, or soft soap? Do you want something that will really clean you well or something that will be better at moisturizing your skin?

Then of course you need to make all your soap in something and you can't use your regular pots and pans unless you are happy having caustic materials and essential oils over your next stir fry.

In the next sections we're going to look at some of the things to consider when choosing your tools and ingredients.

Chapter 3: Soap Making Processes

Modern day has brought us many benefits such as the internet, digital TV, and cell phones but when it comes to our health and skin care, we are swamped with everyday commercials advertising all sorts of skin care products which are filled with chemical additives, detergents, fillers, petroleum, high animal fat content, and irritants that are very often the reason for dry skin, rash, and other irritations. No matter how much we try to minimize toxins that enter our body daily, one thing we can never be sure about is how good or bad the artificial skin care products are offered on the market today. Commercially produced bars tend to be glycerin free which is what makes your skin so dry and in desperate need for so many moisturizing lotions. This is why more and more people decide to make their own skin care products in the comfort of their home. Natural homemade soaps are becoming more and more popular every day and the results on our skin, according to many statements, are priceless. Once you experience all the benefits of a natural product on your skin, you will find it difficult to go back to artificially masked soap promoted as a healthy soap for you and your family.

In this book, we will go through different processes of making soap at home, and you will be able to decide which process is the best for you. Hopefully, you will then choose to make your own soap which will treat your skin the way it deserves to be treated.

Before you start   making your   own soaps, you need   to first   gain an understanding of the different processe s in making them. This will help you find out what process is easier for you. It is recommended that you start with the simple soap making processes first, just to reinforce the idea that you can do this, and maintain your interest in the craft.

There are five soap making processes which allow you to make soap in the comfort of your own home. The processes and their steps are discussed below.

Melt and Pour (M&P) Process

Melt and pour soap making is the easiest way to make soap. Even though it is often called the "cheat" process, it can help you make a very simple and easy first step in your endeavor to make soaps at home. The difference between Melt and Pour and the Cold Processes is that in M&P you do not need to be involved in the preparation of the base, which is why many people find it much "cleaner" and a safer way of making homemade soaps. This process is basically the "artistic" one that provides you freedom in combining scents, colors, and shapes without so much effort. In reality, you are not really making soap using this process. This process only allows you to add scents and colors, making shapes out of a melted pre-made clear soap base which can be a very fun hobby for the entire family. However, precaution is still necessary, especially around small children while handling the hot liquid base that can generally be over 120 degrees.

Even though many people do not pay attention when it comes to choosing the pre-base for their melt and pour soap, pre-base for this process should be a basic soap made through saponification without any additives. This process can be a very fun and easy experiment at home. The most important thing when creating your skin care products should be finding the right natural soap base. Making sure to buy completely natural and synthetic-free pre-base will allow you to experience real skincare benefits of your newly made soap. This is the reason you should buy only a natural and glycerin soap base which acts as a very moisturizing and healing product for your skin.

Once you have found your perfect base, the next step should be preparing all the necessary supplies and ingredients. For this method, you should prepare a large, heat resistant, measuring cup which should hold at least 1 liter; a double boiler or a microwave; sharp knife and wooden spoon, melt and pour base; soap making dye and mold; and, of course, your choice of essential oils and skin care nutrients.

Once you get everything prepared, there are only four steps in M&P soap making:

First, you need to melt the soap in a double boiler or a microwave (make sure to cut solid soap base into small chunks for easier melting). Second, when it has completely melted, measure your fragrances or essential oil and put in a small bowl then add a coloring you desire. Make sure you use soap and skin-safe dyes or natural colorants. Add the melted soap base and stir to blend the fragrance and color. Avoid stirring too hard, or you will have bubbles in your soap. Once you have completed these two steps, slowly pour the soap into the mold. Your soap should be ready and hard enough to remove from the mold in a few hours. The fourth step is stamping the soap, which is optional.

Cold Process (CP)

Making soap is a process that demands a lot of time, effort, and patience but results with a great product that will be extremely useful for your family, friends, and anyone you decide to share it with. The basic way of making soap from scratch at home is "cold process." As the name says for itself, no heat is added to the soap during this process, except what is needed to melt the oils.

The cold process is the easiest and most popular way of making soap from scratch, but it involves the curing stage which makes the process longer. The most important thing when it comes to making soap from scratch is that you are always in control of the ingredients that go into your soap. In this process, you will create the soap base. There are two basic ingredients in the CP process. These are your base oils, which will be discussed later, and a chemical called lye.

The main thing before starting with a process is to choose your recipe. If this is your first time making soap or you think you are still at the "beginner" level, I would suggest you to choose one of the simple recipes to start with. After you succeed in making your first soap you will be able to experiment and make any soap you would like.

The next step is to make sure you have all the necessary equipment, ingredients, and materials. This step is very important as it will help you in the organization and make the entire process much easier. It is very important to be aware that since you will be working with lye, you should wear your safety equipment during the entire process.

Now you need to measure the water and put in a heatproof glass jar, Pyrex measuring cup, heavy duty polypropylene plastic or stainless steel container and add the lye. Once this step is finished, make sure to put this container somewhere safe and label it so there is no possibility that someone might mistakenly drink it. Weighing of all the ingredients should be done with a digital scale, including liquids.

Previously measured solid oils need to be carefully added one by one into your soap pot. It is best to add a bit more now because you can't add extra later. When you are finished with mixing your solid oils in the soap making pot, place the pot on the stove on over medium heat. Gently stirring and monitoring the temperature constantly are highly recommended until all the solid oils are finally melted.

After your solid oils are melted, add the liquid oils to the soap pot. Liquid oils should be at room temperature which will bring the overall temperature in the soap pot down.

This step requires great attention so make sure you have all the soap making additives ready and within reach. During this step, you will add the lye-water mixture to the soap pot.

Use the digital scale and measure out your lye. While measuring, make sure you wear gloves and goggles. To avoid the "lye" volcano, add the lye to cold or room temperature water. Make sure to always add lye to water, not the other way around. Add the lye-water solution to the melted oils once they cool.

Once the lye-water mixture is added to your melted oils, you will instantly see the reaction of oils which will make the oils turn cloudy. You will need to move the pot steadily, take the electric mixer (you can stir by hand as well, but this method will take you a much longer time) and stir the mixture at intervals of 3- 5 seconds, you will be able to see the soap mixture finally begin to come together. Keep blending until everything is completely mixed together.

When you notice that the mixture of your future soap is completely blended, slowly add the fragrance or essential oils to it. Make sure to do this before the mixture becomes too thick. Once the fragrance or essential oils are added, continue stirring using the spoon. At the end, use your hand mixer just once more to make sure that everything is well mixed and add the color of your choice. The most popular colors for homemade soaps will be discussed later in the chapter, but this is your time to play and decide how your custom-made soap will look. There are two ways of adding the color to the mixture. If you prefer your soap to be one color, then simply add the colorant to the pot and stir. A very popular effect in Cold Process soap making is the "swirl effect." If you want your soap to look swirly, ladle one cup of the soap mixture into a measuring cup and simply add the colorant to it. Slowly pour the colored soap mixture into the pot with the rest of it and make sure not to stir it too much, otherwise, the color will blend, and you will have a single-color soap.

The very the last thing you should do before leaving your soap to the saponification process is to pour the raw soap into the mold and evenly spread it out. Smooth it out with a spatula and gently tap your mold on the counter top.

This way you will be sure that there are no air bubbles or trapped air in your soap.

Choose a safe and warm place for your soap and leave it with a towel around it or over the mold to help to keep it warm, so the reaction stays strong. It usually takes about 24 hours for your soap to harden but wait for at least two days before taking it out of the mold and slicing.

Carefully wash everything you have used in the soap making process. Slice your soap depending on your personal preference and put it aside to cure. Saponification is the process that usually takes several days, after that, you can use your soap. However, it is recommended to be patient and wait at least 4- 6 weeks. This way you will be sure your soap will not fall apart during the first use. Cold process is known for the long period of "curing" but is very popular as the soaps are much smoother, easier to shape and color as you wish.

Hot Process (HP)

Hot process is a quicker way to make soap. It used to be called the kettle process.

The Hot Process is very like the Cold Process because you use the same base recipes. The Hot process, however, requires the heat source to bring the soap into the gel phase. While making your soap with the Cold process there is as much as one hour during which you do not have to pay attention to the cooking itself. The Hot Process requires your full attention all the time so make sure you have no other obligations before starting this process. Before you decide to make your soap using the Hot process you need to be aware it will take at least two hours (especially if this is your first time) without any distractions. It is highly recommended not to start the process while children or pets are in same room.

The first few steps in Hot Process are the same as in Cold Process. Before you start with a process, you need to choose your recipe. The easier the recipe you choose, the easier your first attempt at making your soap with this process will be. If you are still in the phase of learning and researching about this method, choose the simple recipe until you become more confident. Once you successfully make your first soap, you will want to try again. When you get confident enough in your soap making skills, you will be able to use all the ingredients you want, including making your own recipe without limiting yourself.

As we already stated in Cold Process, accurate measuring is very important so take your time and measure all the additives, including the essential oils you are going to add at the end.

Once you measured the water, carefully measure the lye as well. Pour the lye into the water slowly and stir it gently till the lye crystals are completely dissolved.

The next step should be easy, especially if you have already tried making soaps using Cold Process. Put your solid oils together and melt them at low temperature. Once the solid oils are completely melted, add the liquid oils and stir it together. You do not need to cool the oils before adding the lye- water mixture.

This step is what makes Hot Process a little bit more difficult than the Cold one. At this phase, you will need to mix the lye-water with oils. Start pouring slowly a thin stream of the lye solution into the pot with oils. Use the whisk or hand mixer while stirring the mixture strong and steady. If you are not using a whisk but are using a hand mixer, make sure to repeatedly combine a pulse for a few seconds with stirring, in intervals.

Once the mixture reaches a thick consistency, you can immediately add the colorant. Adding the colorant at this phase should be only be done if you want your soap to be one color, otherwise, if you want to experiment with colors and swirls in your soap, add the colorant later. Please note that experimenting with colors and swirls in the hot process is much more difficult than when using the Cold Process so do not get upset if your first soap does not have the color you wanted.

You have already put a lot of effort into making your first soap and seeing the final product, no matter the shape or color, it should make you feel satisfied. After few attempts, I am sure your soap will be just as you wanted it to be, perfect!

Even though it will take you more time and attention while using this process for making your soap and the soap might not look as perfect as the one using Cold Process, the advantage of this process is that you can use your soaps immediately after slicing them, without having to wait for weeks to cure.

Cold Process/Oven Process (CPOP)

This process is a new method of soap making at home. Think about it as a bridge between Cold Process and Hot Process in soap making.

The entire recipe and procedure are the same as in Cold Process so pouring it into molds is very easy. The best mold for this process might be the silicon ones which is heat- resistant. After you followed all the Cold Process steps and poured your mixture into the mold, pre-heat the oven and turn it off as soon as you place your mold in it. Close the oven door and leave it at least overnight so the water can evaporate.

It will take your soap another 24 hours before you can slice it into bars once you remove it from the oven. It might take your soap bars a couple of weeks to completely cure, but generally, the soap can be used immediately after slicing.

The disadvantage of this soap making process is that this is not the perfect process to use if you want to have a nice smell to your soap. Essential oils usually evaporate using the higher temperatures so you might end up disappointed when losing some of the nice scents of your soap. On the other hand- this is a very easy way to make your all natural soap!

Milling

Soap milling is also very often called French milling. This is not the actual process of soap making but a method of enhancing an already existing soap. It creates a smoother soap that resembles the texture of a commercialized bar soap.

This method is used as an improvement to your carefully made Cold Process soap.

During the milling process, you are encouraged to use a variety of healing and cleansing ingredients enriching your soap.

To start, you will need unscented and natural soap, hot water and essential oils, herbs or any other ingredients you choose to add to your soap.

The next thing you should do is to grate the soap and add some water (approximately ½ cup of water per 100 grams) and stir it well.

Place your mixture on low temperature and gently stir until the soap is melted and entirely mixed with water. Once you get the perfect mixture, you should remove it from the heat and add all the ingredients except the essential oils and keep stirring.

As we have already mentioned, essential oils do not react to heat very well and adding them to this phase might result by causing them to evaporate.

Once you cool the mixture by stirring you are ready to add the essential oils. Stir it while adding oils and spoon your mixture into the mold. Put it aside to harden and dry.

All you have to do now, once your soap bars are hard and dry enough is to unmold your soap and leave it for few weeks on waxed paper.

This soap can last for a very long time, but some scents may become less strong within a few months.

Chapter 4: Diy Soap 101

Before you get started on your soap making experience, you are going to need to arm yourself with plenty of information. This chapter will get you started.

Soap Making Basics

Once you understand these basics of soap making, everything else will make much more sense!

Lye is important!

All soaps are made from lye. There are many different varieties of lye, from chemically created lyes to those that are naturally made from ashes. Depending on whether or not you want to use all organic materials in your soaps, you may want to choose a supplier who makes lye the natural way, with no chemicals involved.

No matter how you choose to get your lye, you will need it for any variety of soap you plan to make!

Oils come next!

Think of your soap as a cooking recipe. You wouldn't want to put olive oil in a sweet baked dish, since it would change the flavor and consistency of the food you are trying to create. The same is true of soaps. Depending on the variety of oil you choose to use, the fats in that oil will react differently with your lye base, creating unique, individual varieties of soap.

Get your measurements right!

Soap making recipes rely on the weight of their ingredients. This means that it is easy to understand what the correct ratio of your ingredients should be. To scale up or down the recipe, you can use a lye calculator or simple multiplication.

Soap Making Methods

Melt & Pour

This method of soap making is great for the beginner who doesn't want to run too many risks or get too involved. However, it isn't very exciting and doesn't leave much room for creativity. Craft stores generally sell the "soap base" used in this process, which is just an uncolored, unscented block of soap that has been made ahead of time. Some melt & pour sets also come with their own soap molds to pour the soaps into.

With this method, you only need a microwave-safe bowl, plastic or stainless steel spoons, measuring spoons, the desired oils or fragrances you want to add to the soap, and of course the soap base and molds.

It is very simple to use the melt & pour method. All you have to do is melt the soap base in the microwave, add the oils and fragrances of your choosing, pour the soap into the molds, and let it harden.

This is the easiest way of making soap, but since you aren't really making it from scratch, it isn't the same as homemade soap. You don't have any control over the ingredients used in the soap base, and most of these bases have had chemicals added to them by the manufacturers. It is impossible to make a truly natural or organic soap by this method.

Cold Process

Cold Process soap making is generally the way most people begin their adventures in creating their own soaps. It is much more unique and original than melt and pour soaps, but it is also very easy. This makes it the best choice for beginners who want to accomplish the entire task of soap creation on their own.

Cold processing is achieved by first heating your base oils (not your fragrance oils) in a pot on the stove to approximately 100 degrees Fahrenheit. Once they have reached the desired temperature, a lye and water mixture is slowly added and blended with an immersion blender until it reaches trace. At this point, the soap can be tampered with to your liking—feel free to experiment with fragrances, color, and other additions. Just be sure to add them all in slowly and watch for seizing! When this step is complete and your soap is fully blended and ready to go, simply pour it into the mold to let it cure.

You can read more details about cold process soap making in Chapter 4 of this book.

Hot Process

The Hot Process method of soap making is a little bit more difficult and complicated than cold process, because it includes a few more steps. However, many soap makers prefer to use this method, since the soap that it creates has more of a rustic aesthetic than cold processed soap does. While it is not recommended for your first try, there's no reason to be afraid of hot processing!

Hot processing begins the same way as cold processing: the oils are heated and the lye and water mixture is added to them and mixed to trace. This is the point when the processes begin to differ. In hot processing, the goal is to speed up the saponification process and force the mixture to turn into a gel very quickly. In order to do this, heat must be added to the mixture, which is usually done by cooking the soap in a slow cooker.

Only after the soap has saponified can you mix in your fragrances, colors, and other additives. After they have been incorporated, you can pour the soap into your mold and leave it for 24 hours to cure.

You can find more information about hot process soap making in Chapter 5 of this book.

Rebatching

This method is generally used to correct mistakes that are made during the process of soap making, such as a major seize. Simply put, to rebatch soap, you first create an initial batch that you will then chop or grate into small pieces to use in repeating the process. Another term for rebatching is reprocessing. This can create what some people refer to as "milled soap."

Other than to correct mistakes, rebatching can also be used to add ingredients to the soap mixture that may react poorly to the lye. Some additives and fragrances won't survive the initial soap making process, so they must be added later in a rebatch.

Before You Get Started

• Safety first! Remember to always be careful and use proper equipment when you are working with your soaps. This will go a long way in keeping you and your household safe during your soap adventures.

• Gather your ingredients and equipment before you start working, and double check to make sure you have everything within easy reach. Some parts of the soap making process absolutely cannot be left unattended. While you are checking, be sure all of your equipment is clean and free of any damage.

• Put down newspapers, tarp, tablecloths, or other coverings to keep your workspace safe from spills. Lye can damage countertops if you don't protect them!

• Label your ingredients carefully, and keep dangerous ones out of reach of children. Make sure your whole family understands what you will be doing, and that you will need some time to yourself to finish the process safely.

• Be sure you understand what you're doing, too! Read through this book completely, and if you need clarification on any step of the process, don't be afraid to check out other online sources or library books. The more you understand, the less likely you are to make mistakes!

• Wear protective eyewear, such as goggles, to keep lye fumes or accidental splashes from your eyes.

• Wear rubber gloves throughout the entire process, not just when working with lye. You can burn your skin with raw soap as well.

• Wear old clothing, or protect your clothing with an old apron or other similar item.

• For lye spills, keep white vinegar handy. Vinegar can neutralize lye and will make the spill less destructive.

• Take your time, go slowly, remember to follow every step carefully, and never ever leave your work unattended!

Chapter 5: Commercial Soap

Commercial Soaps

A larger percentage of the population hold the perception that bar soaps, one of the oldest cleanser in the world, is harmless. As opposed to popular opinion, modern-day commercial soap is filled with synthetic chemicals that brings along with it different health risks. Several of the products we all use for hygiene—body washes, facial cleansers, and soaps—might actually be causing more harm than good. One of the major means through which the body get the nutrient apart from eating is through the skin – trans-dermally. The skin is the largest organ in the body with an average of 22 square feet and 60 per cent of the substances that are applied on the skin eventually seeps into the bloodstream. This skin which acts as a semipermeable membrane gives us the chance to absorb minerals and vitamins, but, unfortunately, the skin also absorbs harmful chemicals that are put on the skin. Chemicals present in most commercial soaps are not to be taken lightly, they can promote allergies, cause hormonal imbalance, promote reproductive problems and increase the likelihood of certain cancers. With debilitating side effects such as these, it is imperative to pay closer attention to the things we apply on the skin.

These are some of the most prominent health effects that different researches have linked to ingredients present in most commercial, personal care products:

Sinus issues;

Escalating Asthma;

Tiredness;

Nausea;

Dizziness;

Headaches;

Cough and Sore throats;

Hives, Dermatitis, Rashes, Eczema;

Irritations to eyes, lungs mouth, eyes;

Tightness in the chest;

Breath Shortness.

You should know right now that the people in the health sector are not regulating the meaning of the word "natural" in soaps that are tagged as natural, this makes it quite easy for commercial soaps to claim to be natural while in actual facts, large scale producers are making use of synthetic chemicals that will be discussed in subsequent paragraphs. Also, this chapter will give insights into a recommendation for a cleanser that is truly an all-natural brand of soap that is best for taking care of the skin.

Potentially Risky Synthetic Compounds

Although there are several kinds of chemicals of interest in the commercial soap, there are four synthetic compounds present in commercial soaps that require the most attention:

Parabens;

Triclosan;

Fragrance;

Sodium Lauryl Sulfate (SLS).

The majority of the commercial bar soaps, whether in liquid and other forms in the present-day market are mostly made up of these and harmful chemicals.

Parabens

These ingredients work by mimicking estrogen, this means that once it is used on the skin, parabens make its way into the bloodstream, and the body is deceived into thinking that it is estrogen. When the body is made to believe that the level of estrogen is abnormally high as a result of these hormone disrupters, the body is forced to react in certain ways such reducing muscle mass, and this can also lead to early puberty, an increase in fat deposits and causing reproductive issues in both women and men. Parabens act as a preservative in most commercial soaps. Health practitioners have advised people to avoid preservatives in the food they consume, and it only makes sense to avoid preservatives when it comes to body and skincare products. Since parabens cause hormonal imbalance by mimicking estrogen in the body, it can increase the risk of breast cancer in some women. This can also lead to health issues for young children as a result of this.

Triclosan

This chemical is usually present in antibacterial soap. Recent researches have proven that triclosan is actually encouraging the presence and growth of bacteria that are resistant to antibiotic cleansers. It also forms dioxin, a carcinogen that was discovered in high levels in the breast milk of humans. The endocrine system suffers from the disruptive behaviour of dioxins; it also has a negative effect on thyroid functions. Did you know that the primary toxic component in Agent Orange! The first antibacterial liquid hand soap that enjoyed commercial success in 1995 is dioxin. This liquid hand soap claims to be ten times more powerful at removing disease-causing agents than the regular liquid soap. Several years after these events, antibacterial soaps have grown to become an industry that generates 16 billion dollars annually when shampoo, toothpaste, dishwashing agents and other types of household cleaners are added to the "antibacterial" list. In recent years, 30% of bar soap and 75% of liquid soaps in the United States are antibacterial cleansers, and they all contain triclosan. Scientist discovered in a research that was published in March 2004 that people who used antibacterial cleaners and soaps showed allergy and allergy symptoms just as often as people that only use regular soaps and cleansers, this simply means triclosan filled antibacterial soap gives little or no protection when compared to regular soaps against diseases causing agents. Present studies are indicating that if the popularity of anti-bacterial soap continues to experience meteoric growth, disease-causing germs could evolve and become more resistant; thus we could be saddled with super germs that will be hard to get rid of.

What the Antibacterial Soap Makers Do Not Tell You

The triclosan used in the production of antibacterial soaps cannot differentiate between bad and good bacteria. But the human body needs good bacteria to survive, as they help protect the body against harmful, bad bacteria. Triclosan will make our immune systems increasingly exposed to the continuous use of antibacterial soaps. In the early stages of childhood, children should be exposed to certain bacteria in bids to grow and strengthen their immune systems, but the major target market of antibacterial soap producers is parents with young children. Therefore, children whose immune system is not exposed to these common bacteria -- because these bacteria have been removed by antibacterial cleanser or soap are more likely to develop an allergy or asthma.

Several studies have also shown that the continuous use of triclosan:

Kills the cells on the skin;

Makes the skin dry;

Can escalate skin problems like psoriasis and eczema;

It does not curb most illnesses, since flues, colds, and more are viral health condition (antibacterial only deals with bacteria, not viruses);

Dioxin, a compound that is highly carcinogenic may be formed during the production process of triclosan, and this makes it a likely contaminant.

Finally, triclosan has now been discovered in the breast milk of 3 out of 5 women. It is also one of the most commonly found compounds in streams, rivers, and other water bodies, usually with a high-level concentration and is quite harmful to different types of algae. This can disrupt aquatic ecosystems.

Sodium Lauryl Sulfate (SLS)

Sodium Lauryl Sulfate (SLS) is one for the most harmful compounds that can be found in almost all personal care product that is on sale, including shampoo, soap, conditioner, and cosmetics. SLS is the most common chemical in car soaps, engine degreasers, garage floor cleaners, and personal body-care products, and it is an anionic surfactant. These chemicals are used for the production of bubbles and lather in soap. Sulfates are dangerous chemicals because it removes the natural oils of the skin, thus increasing the permeability of the skin surface. SLS also acts as an irritant to people that have eczema or people with sensitive skin. As a result of SLS lathering ability, it is the substance in the soap that irritates the eyes (especially in little children). I guess this would make it necessary to buy other products after you are "clean" to soothe your already irritated skin. Apart from being an irritant, Sodium Lauryl Sulfate is also hazardous as it has been linked to cancer, endocrine disruption, and neurotoxicity according to certain researches. Anyone that cares about his or her health should avoid the everyday use of products that contain these harmful chemicals.

SLS has been found to be responsible for the following:

Skin, eye, and mouth irritations;

Alteration of the skin membrane;

May be dangerous to the heart, brain, liver, and spleen;

Contact dermatitis;

It compromises the overall integrity of the skin barrier, leaving it open to harmful bacteria to penetrate;

May actually disrupt the functioning of cells;

Can affect the hair follicle, thus leading to hair loss.

People with sensitive skin need to pay more attention to these debilitating side effects because a skin that is sensitive might not be able to deal with the irritation caused by soaps and body care products that contain sodium laurel sulfate. This can be quite frustrating as a product that is meant to help the skin is actually causing skin harm. Although, there is an increase in public awareness about the side effects of "sulfates" in recent years and you will still find them in several products – especially shampoos – that claim to be sulfate-free. There are still several perceptions about the harmful side effects of sulfates, but evidence points out that it is best to avoid the everyday use of products that contain these compounds.

Fragrance

Close to 95% of the chemicals used for the production of fragrances are synthetic compounds that are petroleum-based. But, most of these chemicals did not undergo a safety test. Commercial soap and body care product manufacturers just need to write "fragrance" on the label, and that is all. Additionally, if "unscented" is printed on a product label, there is a higher probability that it contains a masking fragrance. Only products with the mark "without perfume" indicates the absence of any type of fragrance. This means, if the ingredient is ambiguous, there is something hidden in the product. Since it not well defined, the term "fragrance" can actually be a mixture of different harmful chemicals they are not telling us, and you'd never find out. It is not a standard requirement by the FDA for companies to mention all the ingredients used for the production of fragrance because the chemicals used for the production are regarded as "trade secrets." Synthetic compounds and cancer-causing toxins such as phthalates (one of the compounds that are used to make fragrances last longer) are hidden under a vague term. Continuous exposure to fragrance has been linked to having a negative effect on the central nervous system and can lead to migraines, allergies and asthma symptoms. Instead of using materials that are natural and beneficial to the body, these commercial soaps expose the skin to several artificial chemicals. It is possible to absorb close to 60% of what comes in contact with the skin. When it enters the skin, these harmful chemicals move through the bloodstream into the sensitive organs in the body. And when we are talking about artificial fragrances, the body can take everything in. With areas that are sensitive in the body such as the genitals taking in over 60% of ingredients. That makes it imperative to be careful when it comes to what comes in contact with your skin.

Why Make Your Own Soap?

Several beauty soaps are not real soap but contain ingredients that can be found in detergent. Also, making your own soap is easy and less expensive when compared to buying soap;

The glycerin is intact when you manufacture your soap yourself;

Making your own soap gives you the chance to pick the kinds of butter and oil that best suit the needs of your skin;

Manufacturing your own soap gives you the opportunity to choose the scent you like;

Soap production brings out your creativity; it is an enjoyable activity and will change the condition of your skin;

Most commercially produced soap is filled with harmful petroleum content and toxic chemicals;

Natural and handmade soaps do not remove natural oils from the skin; it rather helps with the preservation of the skin;

Commercial soap can cause dry and unhealthy skin since the glycerin has been removed and repackage for cream and lotion producers. Glycerin works by pulling moisture from the atmosphere to the skin;

Handmade and natural soaps aid people suffering from skin issues like eczema, psoriasis, and sensitive skin find fast relief after they decided to give handmade soap a try.

Natural Soaps

As a result of the growing awareness about the harmful side effects of a typical commercial soap and body care product, there has been an increase in interest in the making of natural, handmade, soap. This is majorly due to the fact that handmade soap uses natural ingredients during the soap making process. One such ingredient is glycerin – a natural humectant that adds more moisture to the skin. Various commercial soap does not add glycerin to their product, but they sell it as another product to be added to their higher-end creams and lotions. However, the word natural is totally unregulated when it comes to soap and cosmetics as a whole, and I am urging you to be ready whether you are making or choosing a healthy replacement for commercial soaps. Natural soaps can be likened to modern versions of ancient methods that produced soaps by blending alkali solutions with oils of a coconut palm, coconut, and olive. Natural and homemade soaps usually last about twice as long as commercial soap bars, they are extremely soothing and moisturizing. Your skin will enjoy drinking the contents of the soap, moisturizing goodness of handmade soap. If you have a hypoallergenic or sensitive skin, natural homemade soaps are meant when it comes to finding immediate relief. They are also healthy, and natural homemade soaps will help you relax, and pamper yourself and your loved ones. People suffering from dermatitis, eczema, and psoriasis usually react harshly to laundry and other common commercial cleaning products. Most of these commercial cleaners (including laundry detergent) are produced with petrochemicals that are very harsh on the skin and the environment as a whole.

Do you know your skin type?

Here's A Small Test to Explain Identifying Skin Type

Pick a cotton ball and moisten it with alcohol or witch hazel.

Rub the moist cotton with the side of your nose.

Pause for ten minutes.

Repeat the process

Check the last cotton ball, and if it is dirty, you might have oily skin.

The cotton is usually clean for people with dry skin.

Natural Handmade Soaps:

Give the skin a natural moisturizer and conditions the skin;

High in glycerin and no free alkali;

Plant-based Oils such as coconut, palm, and olive is used for production;

Filled with certified organic spices, herbs, grains, and botanical concentrates;

No usage of lab rats;

No animal by-products;

It is not toxic;

Won't leave the skin dry;

Absence of preservatives;

Absence of artificial colours;

Thicker bars mean a longer period of use;

100% organically hypoallergenic;

Absence of Sodium Lauryl Sulfate;

Absence of alcohols, detergents, artificial fragrances, and d-limonene.

Meanwhile, most commercial soaps and body care products:

Leave the skin dry due to the presence of free alkali salts and little or no glycerin content;

Contain the by-products of animals and a higher level of coconut oil;

Contain synthetic preservatives, fragrances, and alcohols;

It does not last long due to high animal fat content and lower density;

It might cause allergies due to chemical composition;

Can pollute the environment;

Toxic;

Remove the natural moisturizers of the skin;

Contain more than 5,000 chemicals;

The glycerin is removed, and fillers are used including synthetic detergents;

Excess alkali can be present in the soap, and this will cause itchiness.

Natural Soap Vs Commercial Soap

As the largest and only external organ on the human body, the skin comes into direct contact with different contaminants every day. On top of the bacteria and dirt that comes in contact with, the skin also readily takes in any compound that is present in the soap you use to clean yourself. The verdict: contrary to popular opinion, maybe commercial soaps are not so perfect after all? Let's do a step by step breakdown of natural soap vs commercial soap.

Main Ingredient Showdown

It is vital to have proper knowledge about the dangerous ingredient before going for commercial soaps and other body care products. The aim of using a bar of soap is to refresh the skin, not to contaminate it with harmful chemicals. Useful trick – if you have a hard time pronouncing the words on the label of the product, put it back on the shelf!

Harmful Commercial Soap Ingredients

Parabens: also referred to as chemical preservatives, these harmful ingredients are present in most commercial soaps and body care products;

Phthalates: known to make cells carcinogenic, this additive is usually used as a 'plasticizer'- a fancy word for the material used for the production of plastic;

Petrochemicals: these are materials made from petroleum; these compounds are not safe for human use because little or nothing is known about the long-term side effects on our health;

Synthetic Perfume: artificial perfume scents are associated with hormonal imbalance and allergies. Also, synthetic materials like perfume can lead to skin issues and can aggravate existing problems like acne;

Artificial Colouring: commercial soaps are filled with artificial dyes that are known to cause illnesses and health issues in humans.

Healthy Natural Soap Ingredients

Healthy Oils: despite popular opinion – oil is actually a vital ingredient when it comes to soap production, especially for people with acne-prone or oily skin. Oils like grapeseed oil, coconut oil, or olive oil aid in the nourishment and moisturizing of the skin bringing it back to its normal PH levels;

Essential Oils: natural soaps with scent are produced with essential oil in bids to produce a natural, harm-free odour;

Oatmeal, Honey, Aloe, etc.: natural soaps are produced with natural materials that are biodegradable that are gotten, produced or harvested in a conscious and safe way;

Unlike the raw materials used for the production of commercial soaps, a consumer can understand the ingredients used for the production of natural soaps and how the body will react to such ingredients.

How It Is Made

Soap producers range from large scale industrial producers to every day do it yourself fanatics. However, the methods employed for the production of soap and the environment where they are produced can have a drastic effect on both the benefits and quality of the soap.

Commercial Soap Production

Mass Produced: the majority of commercial soaps are manufactured by big multinational corporations with factories in different parts of the world. This large scale production leads to a huge amount of industrial wastes that have a massive negative effect on the environment as well as poor living conditions for millions of people across the globe.

Factory-Made: commercial soaps are also produced in batches by machines in big industries – in conditions that are not ideal. Most users are not privy to this information regarding the cleanliness and working conditions of the factories where their soap produced.

Natural Soap Production

Locally Produced: natural soaps are usually produced locally with fresh, locally sourced materials. Natural and homemade soaps benefit their immediate environment financially whilst leaving a very minimal carbon footprint during the course of the production.

Hand-Made: hand-made, organic soaps are gaining more traction due to the fact that it is very easy to make and beneficial to the body. When purchasing handmade soap, consumers have the chance to meet the producers and learn more about the ingredients used for the production of the soap.

Made with Care: if a soap producer is only interested in making financial profits, they are not likely to dedicate time to the production of natural soaps as a result of the higher cost of production for large scale manufacturing. As a result of this, most natural soap lines are produced by people that are concerned about the health of the users and the environment at large.

And the Winner Is

There is only one clear winner between natural soaps and commercial soaps, and the winner is natural homemade soaps!

With these facts stated above, it is not a surprise that people with proper awareness are now switching from commercially produced soaps to natural homemade soaps immediately they see the clear difference in their skin and overall health. By not using artificial materials such as chemicals and perfumes with natural soap, consumers now have the chance to boost their overall health and improve their wellbeing.

For individuals who are really interested in making their own soap, they will most likely discover that buying ingredients in large quantities and online is the best way to reduce the cost of producing your own soap. Producing your own soap is not something that can be seen as a cheap or easy pastime as the initial cost of setting up is more than other hobbies like crocheting or scrapbooking. However, people with any sort of skin issue will soon discover that not only is producing your own soap worth the initial cost of the startup but your skin – and the skin of people around you will also reap amazing rewards from what could easily be a new hobby.

Chapter 6: What Goes Into Soap?

Ingredients, ingredients, ingredients

As you definitely know, the significant fixings that you will require so as to make soap are fats, oils, and lye. In the event that you need to take your soap up a score you can include aroma, shading, as well as spices to make a sumptuous bar.

Fats and oils

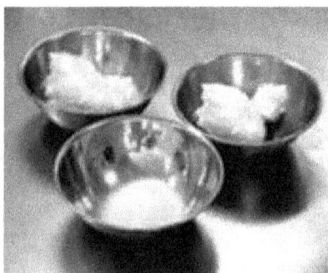

How about we hang out first. The fats and oils utilized in soap are otherwise called the soap base. The main alternative is to purchase fat from a butcher and render it yourself at home. Delivering is the way toward softening the fat and eliminating any muscle tissue or different contaminations so you are left with a smooth material that won't ruin. The delivered fat from pig is called grease. This is a delicate, smooth white substance. The delivered fat from sheep or bovines is called fat and is a hard, coarse strong. On the off chance that you need to deliver your own fat you will require:

3-5 pounds of fat that is hacked (little) or ground

Large pot

Water

Salt

Sieve or Colander

Large bowl

Large spoons

Potato masher

When you have the entirety of your fixings, set them out in an all around ventilated zone as delivering fat is a truly foul cycle. In the event that you have a side burner on your barbecue, do this outside. The family will bless your heart. At the point when you are prepared to begin, follow these means:

Put the little bits of fat into a major pot and add simply enough water to cover it.

Add 1 tablespoon of salt for each pound of fat to the pot.

Turn the warmth on and bring the blend up to a low bubble.

Simmer the fat on a low warmth for 20-30 minutes.

Use the potato masher to push down the fat and accelerate the cycle a little by pressing more oil out.

When you are left with generally seared meat and cartilage in the pot you can kill the warmth.

Caution-you should be exceptionally cautious while doing this following stage. Take the pot off the oven and pour the substance of the container through a colander or strainer and into an enormous bowl. This is best done in the sink.

You will be left with all the solids in your colander and all the fluid in the bowl.

Set the solids aside.

10. Peer into the bowl and you will see a layer of water on the base and the liquefied fat on the top.

11. Cool the fluid to room temperature and afterward move it into the fridge to remain for the time being.

12. In the morning, take the bowl out. You will see the fat or fat has framed a white circle on head of the water.

13. Using a blade or fork, eliminate this plate and put the pieces into a bowl.

14. Dispose of the remainder of the fluid. Remember that it might stop up your sink so unloading it into the fertilizer heap or the patio is a smart thought.

15. If you made fat, clear off as a great part of the free fat particles on it as you can. Run it under cool water to ensure it is totally spotless.

16. Store the fat or fat in the cooler until it is soap setting aside a few minutes.

In the event that utilizing creature fat doesn't sound engaging, it is totally adequate to utilize a vegetable base. This is extremely normal and an assortment of vegetable oils and shortenings can be found at the nearby staple or regular food store. Normally utilized soap bases are olive oil, shea margarine, cocoa spread, and coconut oil. Olive oil is known for being delicate and is likely the most mainstream base. Shea margarine is delicate and ultra-saturating settling on it a decent decision for soap that will be utilized by somebody with dry skin. Utilizing cocoa spread will add immovability to your soap. Coconut oil will create a hard soap with bunches of air pockets in the foam when it is utilized. Other, more uncommon, fats and oils are jojba, palm, sunflower, sweet almond, castor, chocolate, avocado, and cottonseed oil.

There is one final thing to know about with respect to fats and oils. At the point when you begin digging into plans, you will see that some will allude to "superfattened" or "supperfattening" soap. This alludes to including extra transporter oil into your blend. Close to two extra tablespoons are regularly included.

Lye

The following fixing that is required is an antacid. Lye is a basic substance otherwise called burning pop or sodium hydroxide. It is utilized for some, reasons including broiler purging, food relieving and channel opening. Be cautious when working with lye. It is an acidic substance truly fit for consuming, eroding, or devastating living tissue.

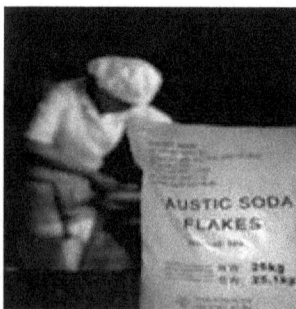

Lye can be bought at a home improvement shop. Be certain that what you buy is 100% sodium hydroxide or harsh pop. You may discover it with stove cleaners or channel openers. It comes in a few structures including chips, pellets, microbeads and coarse powder. Any of these can be utilized in the soap making measure nonetheless; the most secure structure is believed to be drops. In the event that you have hard water at your home, you might need to consider utilizing refined water when blending your lye for better outcomes. Use care when utilizing and putting away lye as it is harmful and destructive.

Significant security note: Lye ought to be put away in fired, stoneware, glass, or warmth safe plastic holders.

Moisturizers

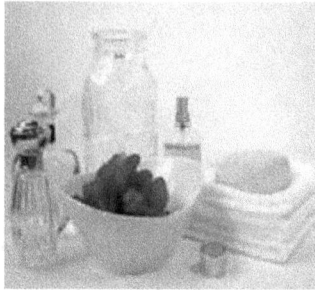

On the off chance that you are hoping to make a truly saturating soap, there are a few fixings you can add to achieve this. You may decide to include additional glycerin. Glycerin is a thick fluid that is dismal and scentless. It is normally delivered during the saponification of fats so you will have just made some glycerin in your soap by joining fat and lye. Glycerin is a humectant implying that it sucks in and ingests water from the air. This makes it extraordinary for keeping the skin saturated. It is water-solvent and has a low harmfulness level.

Shea margarine, coconut oil, almond oil, or nectar can likewise be included for additional moisturization. When looking for shea spread, you will see that there are two sorts accessible refined and crude. Refined shea spread has been prepared at high warmth with synthetic compounds. During that cycle, huge numbers of the advantages of shea margarine are lost. By utilizing a crude shea margarine, you will receive the full rewards from the item. On the off chance that you decide to utilize nectar, include 1 tablespoon for every pound of oil and ensure it is completely blended in before the follow gets excessively thick.

Thickeners and hardeners

Contingent upon the kind of soap you are making and the plan components you will use to accomplish your ideal look, you may decide to add a material to thicken your soap or make it harder. There are a few decisions the first is beeswax. This can be bought at make stores or stores that sell flame making supplies. Beeswax enables the oils in the soap to mix together and turn out to be progressively thick. By making a thicker base, the soap will settle and become harder.

Including salt will likewise build the soap's hardness, from the outset. Observe that salt doesn't expand the hardness of the completed bar, yet it causes the bar to get more diligently quicker. This permits the soap to be unmolded sooner. Salt ought to be disintegrated in water before you add the lye to it. Use about ½ a teaspoon for every pound of oil or fat.

Water alternatives

Despite the fact that it is generally basic to blend lye in with water when making soap, it is unquestionably conceivable to utilize different fluids. Milk is once in a while utilized in soap making to make exceptionally velvety soap. Dairy animals' milk, goat's milk, coconut milk, and even buttermilk can be utilized. It is utilized rather than water in the lye arrangement. A note of alert Milk responds uniquely in contrast to water when blended in with lye because of the sugars that are in it. There is a propensity for the milk to singe as the lye warms up and this could turn the blend earthy colored and foul (not positively). So as to keep this from occurring, the blending cycle can be changed a piece. This methodology can likewise be followed to substitute tea, espresso, or brew for the water in the soap. It is critical to wear security goggles and gloves to do this.

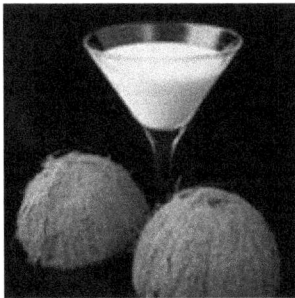

Start with 1/third of the milk in fluid structure and the other 2/third of the milk in a slushy or solidified state.

Prepare an ice shower in your sink.

Add the fluid 1/third of the milk to a tall pitcher or bowl.

Place the bowl in the frigid sink water.

Combine the lye with the milk, adding cold water to the sink to hold the temperatures down varying

Slowly add lye to the milk and mix tenderly. Recall that it is beginning to warm up now.

Go incredibly, gradually permitting the blend to chill off a piece before including more lye.

Start including the slushy or solidified milk to the blend. Be cautious while doing this so it doesn't sprinkle.

Keep including, blending, and mixing until all the milk and lye has been consolidated. Try not to be frightened if the blend turns a brilliant golden shading. It will occur and you should consolidate that into your general soap plan when utilizing milk.

Bubbles, Bubbles, Bubbles

Part of the fun of soap is stirring up an extraordinary foam with huge amounts of air pockets. Two materials, borax and sugar, will assist you with achieving the objective of making foamy soap.

Borax won't just assistance the soap make truly incredible bubbles, it additionally fills in as a disinfectant. You can discover borax in stores, as a rule in the clothing soap segment. By and large, one tablespoon of borax is utilized for each pound of soap base.

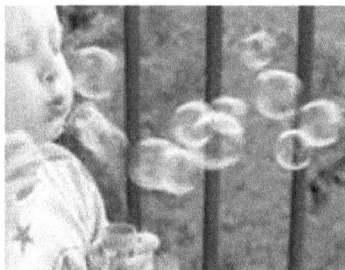

Sugar will likewise expand the measure of foam and air pockets. One approach to add sugar to soap is to altogether disintegrate it in water before including the lye. Another approach to do it is to take a touch of the water you have weighed for use in your lye arrangement and add ½ to one teaspoon of sugar for every pound of oil or fat. Totally disintegrate the sugar, utilizing warm water may help with this. Include the arrangement when your soap is at the follow stage before you include your aroma. The last strategy for adding sugar is to make a syrup by consolidating two cups of sugar with one cup of water and gradually warming the blend. Mix until all the sugar is broken down. Include 1/2 to one teaspoon of this basic syrup to your soap at follow, before including aroma. Know that including sugar can increase the temperature of the soap during the gel process so be extra careful when handling.

Botanicals

Spices and different botanicals are normally added to soap blends to give the soap recuperating properties, shading, as well as scent. A few of these spices can be developed in a nursery and dried. This is a reasonable method to get these fixings and is an incredible selling point if you are anticipating selling the soap that you make. If you have a nursery, plant a little segment of "soap botanicals" or make a smaller than expected indoor nursery if you like. The accompanying botanicals are anything but difficult to develop and are incredible for utilizing in soap making:

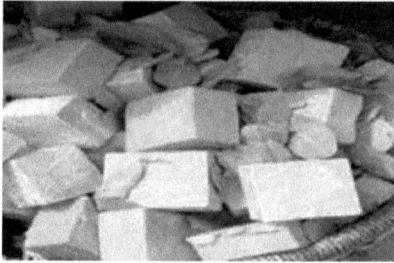

☐Calendula

☐Comfrey

☐Lavender

☐Mint

☐Basil

☐Rosemary

☐Peppermint

☐Spearmint

☐Lemongrass

☐Chamomile

☐Sage

☐Thyme

At the point when they are prepared, pick the botanicals and dry them preceding utilizing in a soap. If developing spices are excessive, head over to the supermarket, or even better a characteristic food store and buy spices there. We will talk in more insight concerning botanicals later on in this book.

Fragrance

Numerous individuals like a foul soap. There are bunches of choices however regardless of anything else, make a point to pick added substances that are cosmetically sheltered, implying that they won't hurt skin. The rules for skin safe aroma are directed by the Research

Institute for Fragrance Materials and the International Fragrance Association. While picking a scent for soap, you should choose if you will utilize aroma oils or fundamental oils. Fundamental oils are the regular embodiment of a plant. The embodiment can emerge out of leaves, blossoms, bark, berries, roots, needles, seeds, beans, strips, cones, wood, stalks, or different pieces of the plant. A plant's pith is acquired either by refining or communicating it. One explanation fundamental oils are so costly is that it can take several pounds of plant material to make only one pound of basic oil. To make a pound of basic rose oil it takes more than 2,000 pounds of flower petals. Know that even though fundamental oils are common items, they do contain normally happening synthetics that are not really alright for the skin. Aroma oils are falsely made aromas. They contain synthetic compounds, some normal plant or creature items, and manufactured scent.

The manufactured scent was concocted in the last part of the 1800s and has gotten well known. The two sorts of the scent will last around 1 year when put away inside a dull glass in a dim, cool room. We will discuss scents again in a later part.

Color

Color is a significant part of making soaps look engaging and attractive to utilize. There are numerous kinds of dirt, mineral colors, micas, and flavors that are affirmed by the Food and Drug Administration for use in beautifiers. Similarly, as with scent, you should pick a shading that is skin protected and endorsed for makeup. A few people mess with utilizing colored pencils and kool help. Even though these are fruitful in giving your soap shading, they are not affirmed as being alright for your skin. Try not to utilize food colorings, texture colors, light colors, paints, or pastels as these have not been affirmed for restorative use. Manufactured hues were found in the nineteenth century. These hues were called Tar Colors and were utilized in food and beautifiers. These fabricated materials were discovered to be hurtful to people and a considerable lot of them were restricted when the US Congress presented the Food and Drug Act in 1906. In 1939, engineered colorings were separated into 3 classifications: FD&C colorants which can be utilized in food, medications, and beautifying agents, D&C colorants which are colors and shades that are viewed as protected in medications and makeup, and External D&C Colorants which are not utilized in food, since they are harmful, yet permitted to be utilized on the skin and in beautifiers. Remember that albeit External D& C colorants are permitted in beautifying agents, they may not genuinely be protected as the skin can retain poisons from substances applied to it.

Chapter 7: Best Homemade Soap Recipes

12. Ready for challenges!

* Melt and pour process

What better way to surprise your friends than with a beautiful and hydrating homemade soap bar? With only three ingredients, this soap is a real pleasure to make, but a much greater pleasure to use. Lemon essential oil ensures you are refreshed and energized, so you can go through the day with a smile on your face.

You need 1 1/2 cups Shea Butter Soap Base, Dried Lemon zest of 4 lemons and 5 drops Lemon Essential Oil.

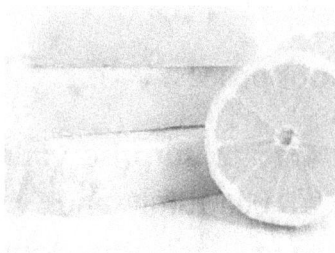

13. Ideal for coffee lovers

*Melt and pour process

Anyone who enjoys the smell of coffee will also enjoy using this soap. This Coffee soap is great for taking a shower in the morning since it will wake up your senses.

You need 1.5 lbs Goat's Milk Soap Base, 1 Tsp of Almond Oil, 1 Tbs. of fresh ground coffee, and 1 Tsp of Fragrance (Coffee or Cinnamon).

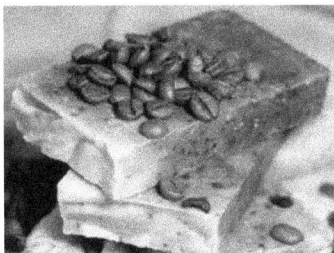

14. Gentle and Soft

*Melt and Pour method

I always struggle to keep my hands moisturized; so if the same goes for you, you can make this Sweet Almond and Poppy seeds soap. You need 2 lb. blocks Shea butter soap base, for hydrating your hands. Also, buy lemon and almond essential oils and add yellow colorant (a few drops). Then, add Poppy seeds.

Poppy seeds are popular for their moisturizing properties. So, with this powerful combination, keeping your hands hydrated and smooth will be a piece of cake.

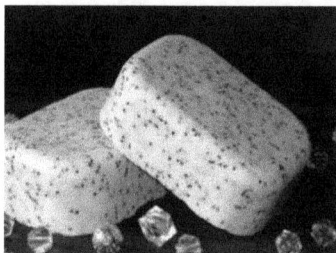

15. Divine beauty

*Melt and Pour method

If you love raspberry and want to enjoy its numerous benefits, you just have to try this Raspberry soap recipe. Within a short time, you get a batch of moisturizing and wonderfully scented soap, perfect for the whole body.

You need 2lb. Aloe soap base, pink soap colorant, and raspberry soap scent. This soap also makes a wonderful gift; so you need to buy a lovely silicone or plastic molds with hearts or flowers.

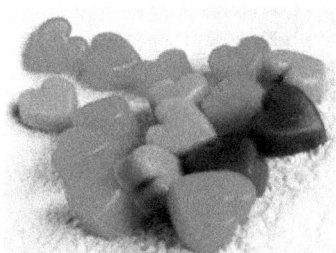

16. To be or not to be?

*Hot process

Here we have another hot process recipe, perfect for those in a hurry. You can give this soap as a gift, or use it right away, without a need to wait for a month to cure. The well-known combination of Olive oil and Coconut oil make this soap a must have in every home.

You need 36 oz. olive oil, 3 oz. castor oil, 6 oz. coconut oil, 6 oz. Lye, 2-4 oz. essential oil of choice, and 12 oz. water.

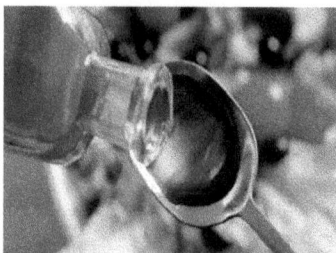

17. Magical and Sensational bath time

*Cold process

You need 90 g Palm oil, 90 g Coconut oil, 30 g Cocoa butter, 90 g Olive Oil, 30 g Castor oil, 46 g Lye, and 100 g water.

Castor oil is a real fighter when it comes to cleaning your pores and fighting bacteria. It will also calm irritated and sensitive skin. Other oils in the recipe will create a powerful yet gentle formula for keeping your skin clean, revitalized and staple, while cocoa butter provides your skin with deep hydration and of course, gives an uplifting smell. This soap is a good choice for anyone looking for a pure way to calm and refresh their skin.

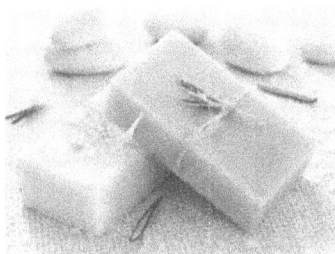

18. Revitalizing and Uplifting

*Melt and Pour method

This simple-to-make soap recipe is ideal for the mornings, whether it is summer or winter. The powerful herbs scent will give you a boost of energy so you will be able to admire the beauty of life throughout the day.

You need Glycerin soap base; 1 tablespoon of each herb additive (mint, basil, rosemary, and orange) and lemon (just make sure to peel off the lemon skin).

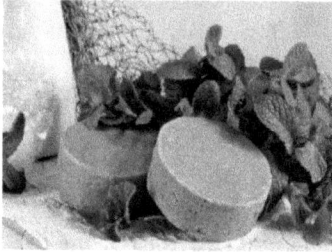

19. Coffee and Chocolate – a piece of heaven

*Cold process

I don't know about you, but I am addicted to coffee and chocolate, and I can't help myself. I even started making soap bars to enjoy that recognizable Mocha scent. Not only that, but taking a shower with Mocha Soap is like a dream come true – it gives me energy, and makes my skin happy. And

I can tell you one thing – when your mornings start with this remarkable combination, your day is bound to be more pleasant.

You need 25% coconut oil, 25% palm kernel oil, 25% palm oil, 12.5% grape seed oil, 12.5% cocoa butter, double strength coffee, and cocoa powder (I put 1 Tsp per one pound of soap, but you can add more if you want darker color).

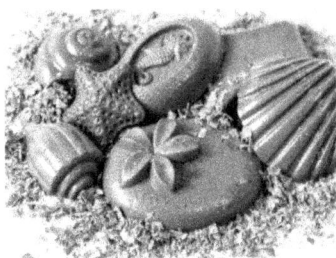

20. Happiness lies in simple things

*Cold process

If you are new to the world of making soap, then this simple recipe will give you a boost of confidence. Be careful when working with the lye, and follow the above-mentioned rules and steps, and everything will be fine. You cannot go wrong with this recipe, so don't panic. It only has Olive oil that will make your skin shine like never before, and of course, will hydrate it. So, if you are looking for a simple

You need 50 oz. (1.5 L) olive oil, 15 oz. (1.5 L) distilled water and 6.3 oz. (178.6 g) lye.

Chapter 8: Equipment

The equipment that you use when making your own soap can be of a variety of shapes, sizes, and qualities, but the one thing that you need to pay special attention to is that you do not use any of this equipment for anything else other than soap making. Equipment that hasn't been washed properly could cause a dangerous situation for people and pets who may come in contact with it. In order to stay on the safe side, always keep the equipment away from where people may find it, and make sure that you don't use a dish washer to wash it; wash it by hand to ensure that none of the substances will come into contact with any of the other dishes that you use for food.

Containers

As you start to create your own soaps and you make your own styles and designs of soap, you will need many different containers in order to bring your imagination to life. However, when you start to choose the kinds of containers that you will be using, there are a few things that you need to keep in mind. For example, the best kinds of containers to use are glass, stainless steel, and plastic. Do not use aluminum bowls because they will react with the lye. When this happens, toxic fumes are released from the container which will enter the soap and infect it with harmful materials.

Thermometer

Depending on which recipe you want to make, you will need to use different temperatures in order to achieve your desired texture and design. In order to do this, you need a very accurate thermometer. You can purchase one almost anywhere, but the best thermometers to use are the ones that are used for tempering chocolate because those will be extremely accurate.

The Blender

No matter what kind of soap you are planning to make, you will always reach a point where you will need to properly mix the lye and the oils in a mixture of your choice. This is not as easy as it may seem. If you were to use a hand whisk to do this, it would take a very long time (perhaps even hours). Remember how we mentioned that the consistency of the soap mixture determines what your finished product will look like in the end? This is where the hand blender comes in handy. It does the job is about 15 to 30 seconds, regardless of what kind of mixture consistency you are looking for. Also, not only will it save you time, it will also greatly increase the quality of your soap products.

Spatulas

You will be using spatulas for a number of different things when it comes to making soap. One of the most important things is to scrape all of the soap from the container when you are putting it into the mold. You really don't want to leave anything behind because it is a loss of money. You will also be using the spatulas to make creative lines and decorations on your soap designs. However, the only spatulas that will properly do the job are silicone spatulas, because the liquid will not stick to them.

A Scale

A good, accurate scale will come in handy at all times when you are making your own soap. Every ingredient needs to be measured properly, even if you are a complete beginner at making your own soap. In order to stick to the highest level of accuracy, the best way to measure ingredients is by weight, which is why a great scale is a must for soap making.

Molds

This is where the best level of creativity will rise. Different molds will allow you to create an almost endless amount of soap designs, and there will always be many different molds to choose from that you can purchase as you become more and more skilled at soap making. However, you need to pay attention to the material of the molds because different molds are used for different kinds of soap making.

Silicone mold: Much like the silicone spoons, silicone molds are also great for beginners, because the soap will not stick to them. You will easily be able to remove the soap from the mold every single time, and silicone is also very easy to clean. Even if you need to heat up the mold, silicone will be able to withstand a fairly high level of temperature.

Wooden molds: These molds are used when you want to make large batches of soap. However, you need to first prep the wood before you are able to use it. This is done by lining the wood with either baking paper or silicone to ensure that the soap mixture will not stick to the edges and that the whole thing will be easier to clean. You can make your own wooden molds as you become more and more skilled in the future so that you can work with your own desired shapes.

Plastic molds: These molds are not the ones that are recommended for use, however, they can be used when making soap with the cold process. If you are going to use plastic molds, you should only use them for soap recipes that are very quick, where the soap will not stay in the mold for a long period of time because it will be almost impossible to clean the mold after use.

The History of Soap Making

In order to inspire you to create your own soap, it is important that we go back to history a little bit in order to learn about the beginnings of soap and how they have affected humanity.

The first time that soap was mentioned in history (to our knowledge) was back in 2,800 B.C. in Babylon. During this period, they used a combination of cassia oil and different alkali salts to make their own soap. The strength of the soap was made depending on whether the salt was intended for human use, washing clothes, or cleaning floors. Ancient Egyptians are especially well-known for their love for bathing, not to mention one of the most famous of them all – Cleopatra.

Europe wasn't as close to soap as the Egyptians were. In fact, it wasn't until the Middle-ages that Europeans actually started to use soap on a frequent basis, and even then, it was usually the rich who had access to soap.

What is the true structure of salt?

Generally, soap is a mixture of salts and oils. The salts are always alkali (or lye), because they are the ones that are able to gently clean the human skin. When it comes to the oils, they can either be animal oils or vegetables oils. However, this was usually in the past. Modern soap design usually relies on more modern oils and scented oils to make the soaps a little more luxurious. However, if you are very new to soap making and you want to test a few batches of your own soap for very little money, then it is a great idea to go back to the traditional, cheap ways of making soap. We will include a few such recipes in this book later on.

Soap got its name because of the chemical reaction that occurs between the lye and the oils, which is known as saponification. The first mixture that comes out of this process is actually glycerin, which later develops into the solid soap texture that we are all familiar with.

Soap has always been only used for external use and as a main cleaning product in the human world. It has never been intended for internal use or in any kind of food, so definitely make sure that you don't bring soap close to food, children, or animals, even if you were the one who made the soap.

Three Different Ways to Make Soap

In general, there are three ways that you can make soap. Which way you use depends on the kind of soap that you are trying to make, the equipment that you have, and also your skill level for making soap. You could choose a single method and stick with it forever, or you can try all three of them and test everything out. However, you will notice that the cold process is the best one for beginners.

Hot Process

This process is very easy to use, but it requires the right equipment and a knowledge of ingredients versus the temperature for the making of the soap. It is easy because you don't really have to worry about the ingredients or how much of them you are adding to the mixture. Even though you still need to maintain a certain balance in what you're doing, the soap will not be ruined if you add more of an ingredient or less of it than you should have.

You need to make sure that you heat the ingredients at the correct temperature for them to compile together into the perfect soap texture, which mostly takes just a good thermometer and some patience. And another great thing about this process is that you can use the soap the very next day. However, as is the case with any of the other processes, it is always better to leave the soap to set for a few days before you use it.

Cold Process

This process is the easiest one to do if you are making soap at home. It is a very easy and fast process when it comes to making soap, and it is also great for the kinds of scents that you want to add to your soap. When you use the hot process, you usually have to be careful with your scents because the heat could damage the strength of your scents and ruin the overall style of your soap.

For this process, you don't have to worry about temperature, but you do have to make sure that your ingredients are at the right proportions and that you mix everything together properly. Also, for the cold process, you will need to wait about a month before you can actually use the soap, but it will definitely be worth the wait.

Melt and Pour Process

This is also another process that is very easy for beginners to use. It is easy because you start the soap making process by actually purchasing the soap base beforehand. Then, with the soap base ready, which has no color or scent, you add your own color and scents to it to make it the kind of soap that you want to use. As soon as this soap design hardens, you can use it the very next day. This is great for beginners to test out their skills, but there is very little to alter in this design because you cannot choose the kinds of oils and salts that go into the mixture.

Chapter 9: Using Soap Base

It is completely understandable if you do not want to start out making soap by messing with lye. Lye tends to scare people away from making soap but that does not have to be the case. If you are afraid to mess with lye but still want to make soap than there is a solution for you. It is making soap by using a soap base.

These are also known as melt and pour soaps but you get to add whatever you want to the soaps to make them your own. You can purchase clear soap base, hemp seed oil soap base, olive oil soap base, aloe soap base and pretty much any other type of base you want. Each of these bases provides different benefits.

These soap bases usually cost about 3 to 4 dollar per pound and you are going to get about 6 bars of soap for each pound of melt and pour you purchase.

The next thing you will want to do is look into purchasing some silicone soap molds. Depending on the molds you purchase as well as where you purchase them from I have seen them run anywhere from less than a dollar to upwards of 70 dollars. If you are just starting out, I suggest you purchase the cheaper molds but if you are going to be running a business selling your soaps it is best to spend the money on the higher prices molds.

Now that you have your melt and pour and your molds you need to figure out what you are going to add into your soap. If you are going to add in essential oils you need to get those, you can all so add in herbs, dried flower petals, oats and even coffee grounds. There really is no limit to what you can add to your soaps. Personally on of my favorite soaps has clay added into it, this is a natural exfoliate and makes the skin super soft. Some people add a bit of sand into their soap while others don't add anything because they prefer a super silky bar.

You can easily embed items in your bars of soap as well, such as a rope or a small toy. To do this, you want to pour half of the soap in the mold when it is time, embed the toy and then pour the other half of the soap.

For this soap you are going to need your scale, a microwave safe bowl, cutting board, metal serving spoon, measuring spoons, a knife and a spray bottle of rubbing alcohol along with the items already mentioned.

First you are going to cut your melt and pour base into 1 inch squares. They don't have to be perfectly one inch or perfectly square, you are only doing this so they melt faster. You will then place the cubes in your microwave safe bowl and microwave them for 30 seconds.

Stir the melt and pour base after 30 seconds and then heat in 10 second intervals stirring after each one until the soap base is completely melted.

After the melt and pour base is completely melted you can then remove it from the microwave and add in all of your additives. This includes any coloring, exfoliates, and essential oils. Make sure you mix very well.

If you find that your soap is starting to set while you are adding in your additives, you can pop it back in the microwave for a few seconds. Now it is ready to pour into your molds. After you have poured the melt and pour into your mold, you need to lightly spray the soap with a bit of rubbing alcohol. This will make sure that there are no air bubbles in the soap.

Now it is time to wait. Set your mold aside and let cool overnight. Once the soap is set you can take it out of the mold. Do not try to speed up the cooling process by placing the soap in the refrigerator because this will ruin your soap.

The great thing about melt and pour soap base is not only do you not have to work with lye, you also don't have to wait four weeks for the soap to age. Once you take it out of the mold you can use it!

If you don't know what type of soap base you really want to work with and you would like to try a few different ones to see which one you like best, you can purchase a melt and pour soap base sampler kit that will come with several different bases.

I suggest you use each one to make soaps with that way you can compare them against each other. You may find that you like a few different soap bases or you may find that different bases work better for the different soaps you make. Making soap is sort of a learn as you go process and you will find not only what soaps work best for you but which ones others like the best if you are selling them.

Once you have made a few batches of soap with the melt and pour soap base you may begin to feel more comfortable with experimenting with lye and making your soaps completely from scratch. If you do not it is completely okay, just because you are using a soap base does not mean you are not making the soaps.

Many people will tell you that using a melt and pour soap base is cheating when it comes to making your own soaps but I think that if you are afraid of using lye and you still want to make your own soaps than go for it.

But I also think that once you give lye a chance you will see that it is not as bad as what many people think. You just have to understand that it is very strong and can be dangerous if it is not handled correctly. In the next chapter we are going to learn how to make another lye soap but we are going to learn the hot process instead of the cold process.

Chapter 10: Choose Your Poison

Which Fats to Use

Making soap is fairly simple - all you really need is a fat and an alkaline in order to create your soap base. Whilst we have a great deal of choice when it comes to which fats to use, the basics will never really change. As long as you get the ratios right, your soap crafting efforts will always be successful.

That said, not all fats are created equal when it comes to soap making. Personally, for example, I prefer a bar of soap crafted from tallow. Other people, however, would prefer soap crafted from a vegetarian source of fat.

Whichever camp you fall in, the choice is yours. Here I will list the most commonly used fats and oils for soap crafting and you can make your own decision.

I will give one caution here - it is tempting to add in as much as you can think of but the best soap bars tend toward the simpler mixtures. Read through this section, try one or two of the recipes and then experiment by adding in other fats if you want to. You may be surprised to learn that more is not always the better option.

Fats

Limit the number of oils that you buy, at least when you are starting out. Tallow, palm oil, olive oil, coconut oil and canola oil are more than enough for you to get your feet wet when you start out. When you learn more and become more practiced at soap crafting, you can start to add in others if you really feel that it is necessary. Personally, I usually use tallow and olive oil and very few other oils because I like a simpler finish. I do believe that society today conditions us to think that choice and complexity is always the better option but this simply cannot always hold true. The beauty of making your own soap is the way that the ingredients almost magically meld together - regardless of how different they seem to be at first.

Tallow

This is rendered animal fat and so not the vegetarian option. I find that a really fine soap can be made from this fat but I do have to admit to being squeamish about rendering the fat myself. That said, I do actually put up with the smell of boiling the fat simply because the soap that results is like nothing you have ever felt before. It is easier to get this to trace than with vegetable oils and makes a nice, long-lasting bar of soap. It is also one of the more affordable options when it comes to fats for soaps.

Find out at the butchers if they will sell you tallow - it does not matter what type of fat, if they will sell you tallow, you are steps ahead. If you cannot get tallow, ask for suet.

Put the suet in a big pot of water over a medium-high heat and allow it to come to the boil. The fat in the suet will rise to the top and the leftover bits of meat will sink to the bottom while the water bubbles away. All that is left to do then is to leave overnight so that the fat hardens and so all that is left for you to do is to scoop off the congealed fat. Turn the fat "brick" over and scrape off any gelatinous material from the underside and your fat is ready for soap crafting. The process is not a particularly pleasant one but it is worth making the effort as I am sure you will agree when you use your first bar crafted from tallow.

For starting out, this is a good option and you can make your soap without incorporating any of the other oils if you prefer and gives a good bar that lathers well and is quite white in color.

Using tallow can be viewed to be historically accurate as well if you consider what soap's origin story is.

Vegetable Oils

Olive Oil (SAP 0.134)

If you are only going to use one of the vegetable oils, it should be olive oil. It is my very favorite of all the vegetable-based soaps and I often blend it with tallow for a luxurious bar that lathers well and lasts well as well.

It doesn't really matter what grade of olive oil you use so select one that suits your pocket, as long as it is pure olive oil that has not been adulterated with other oils. (This is commonly the case with the very much cheaper brands of olive oil.) Your soap is bound to take on a bit of a greenish tint or might even be off-white at best but

I believe that this only adds to the charm. Olive oil has strong anti-bacterial properties and soaps made with olive oil have been known to last decades so this is a really great soap base.

Coconut Oil (SAP 0.178)

Coconut oil is not for everyone. I know that it is touted as a great moisturizer but I find that it is too severe for my sensitive skin. If you are prone to skin allergies or have extremely dry or sensitive skin, do not use coconut oil.

That said, it really does make a great cleanser for normal/ combination skins. It should never make up more than 25% of the total oil content when you make your soap. Coconut bars do not lather as well but do have quite a nice white color to them.

Canola Oil (SAP 0.132)

This is a reasonably fair option if you need to add bulk to a recipe but are following a tight budget. It is a lot better than sunflower oil and should always be chosen in preference to it. It makes a creamy lather and helps to whiten the soap so if you want to color your soap, it is a good option. Use to a maximum of 35% in your recipe overall.

Palm Oil (SAP 0.178)

If you prefer a firmer bar of soap that lathers very well, add in some palm oil. This is an oil that has a firm place in the beauty industry. One caution - If it is used in too high a proportion the bar will be quite brittle so stick to no more than 15% in your recipe overall.

Chapter 11: Soap Recipes You Can Make At Home

Honey Bar

Supplies Needed:

4 ounce coconut oil

4 ounce olive oil

1 ounce canola oil

1 ounce safflower oil

1 ounce sunflower oil

3 ounce beeswax

1.5 ounce lye

3.63 ounce distilled water

3 tablespoons of organic honey

Soap mold

Instructions:

Carefully pour the lye into the distilled water. Stir gently until the lye is dissolved.

Set aside the lye solution and allow to cool.

Warm the beeswax in a pot on low heat until completely melted. Carefully add the first 5 oils one at a time. Make sure that the oils don't get too hot.

Take the pot off the heat.

Carefully pour the lye and water solution into a pot. Stir all the ingredients together.

Using a hand mixer, blend the soap mixture until you get a creamy pudding consistency.

Put the pot back on low heat and let the soap mixture to cook for about an hour or until the mixture turns transparent.

Stir in honey to create swirls.

Pour the soap mixture into the soap molds. Let the soap to dry for 24 hours before cutting them into bars.

Wrap the soaps in wax paper and store in a cool dry area, away from direct sunlight.

Sweetheart Exfoliating Bar

Supplies Needed:

2 cups soap base (shea butter)

4 tablespoons organic honey

4 tablespoons finely ground oatmeal

3 tablespoons chamomile essential oil

Soap mold

Instructions:

Cut the shea butter soap base into small chunks and melt in a heat resistant microwave safe glass bowl.

Set the microwave to 20 second intervals and heat the soap base until it's fully liquefied.

In a separate bowl, mix the finely ground oatmeal with honey until you get a paste.

Allow the melted soap base to cool for 5 minutes before adding the oatmeal paste and chamomile essential oil.

Whisk the soap mixture until you get a thick consistency.

Pour the soap mixture into the mold and set it aside.

Let it harden for at least 5 hours before cutting the soap into bars.

Wrap the soap bars in wax paper. Keep away from direct sunlight.

The Tropics Soothing Bar

Supplies Needed:

1 ½ cup glycerin soap base (shea butter)

¾ cup coconut oil

1 ½ cup fine sand

¾ cup distilled water

Soap mold

Instructions:

Cut shea butter soap base into small cubes.

Put shea butter soap base cubes in a microwave safe glass container and melt for 2-3 minutes in the microwave.

Once the soap base is melted, allow it to cool for 5 minutes.

Stir in coconut oil and distilled water. Add sand and whisk all the ingredients together.

Continue whisking until the soap mixture begins to thicken.

Pour the soap mixture into the mold.

Leave the soap mixture to harden overnight.

Take the soap out of the mold and cut into bars.

Wrap soap bars in wax paper and store in a cool place, away from direct sunlight.

Orange Poppy Seed Nourishing Bar

Supplies Needed:

2 cups soap base (olive oil)

½ cup poppy seeds

1 tablespoon sweet orange essential oil

1 tablespoon dried orange peel

Soap mold

Instructions:

Spread out half of the poppy seeds at the bottom of the soap mold.

Cut the olive oil soap base into cubes.

Put olive oil soap cubes in a microwave safe glass container and melt for around 45 seconds in the microwave. Take the soap base out of the microwave, give it a stir, and put it back into the microwave for a minute until it's completely melted.

Allow the soap base to cool for 5 minutes.

Stir in the sweet orange essential oil. Add the remaining chia seeds and the dried orange peel and whisk it all together.

Mix until the soap mixture begins to thicken.

Pour the orange poppy seed soap mixture into the mold.

Leave the soap mixture to dry and harden for at least 24 hours before taking it out of the mold.

Take the soap out of the mold and cut into bars with a sharp knife.

Store soap in wax paper keep away from direct sunlight.

Asian Sunset Moisturizing Soap

Supplies Needed:

3 cups soap base (castile)

1 cup dried calendula petals

4 tablespoons Ylang Ylang essential oil

Soap mold

Instructions:

Cut the castile soap base into small chunks and put in a microwave safe glass container.

Melt the soap base in the microwave in 30 second intervals until you get a liquefied soap.

Set aside the liquefied soap and let it to cool for 5 minutes.

While waiting for the soap to cool, crumble the dried calendula petals.

Stir in Ylang Ylang essential oil. Add a couple of drops more if you want the scent to be stronger.

Whisk in the dried calendula petals.

Pour the soap mixture into a mold. Allow the soap to dry overnight.

Pop the soap out of the mold and wrap it in wax paper.

Store the soap in a cool dry place, away from direct heat and sunlight.

Night Breeze Soap

Supplies Needed:

2 cups soap base (shea butter)

1 cup clear soap base (aloe vera)

2 tablespoons frankincense essential oil

2 tablespoons eucalyptus essential oil

½ teaspoon blue mica powder

1 tablespoon distilled water

Soap mold

Instructions:

Cut the shea butter soap base into small cubes and put in a heat resistant glass microwaveable bowl.

Heat the shea butter soap base in the microwave in 30 second intervals until it's fully melted.

Set aside the liquefied shea butter soap base and let it to cool for 5 minutes.

Stir in the frankincense essential oil and mix well.

Dissolve the blue mica powder in a 1 tablespoon of distilled water before adding it to the shea butter soap base. Mix well until you get an even color.

Pour the shea butter soap mixture into the mold. Make sure to only fill it halfway.

Cut the aloe vera soap base into small cubes and put in a heat-safe glass microwaveable bowl.

Heat the aloe vera soap base in the microwave until it's fully melted.

Let it cool for 5 minutes before stirring in the eucalyptus essential oil.

Pour the aloe vera soap mixture on top of the shea butter mixture.

1Allow the soap to cure for 24 hours before popping it out of the mold.

1Slice the soap into bars and wrap it in wax paper.

1Keep away from direct heat and sunlight.

Lavender and Charcoal Cleansing Bar

Supplies Needed:

1.5 ounce coconut oil

1.5 ounce olive oil

1 ounce neem oil

1 ounce Grapeseed oil

1.5 ounce castor oil

.85 ounce lye

2.15 ounce distilled water

20 drops lavender essential oil

1 ½ tablespoon activated charcoal powder

Soap mold

Instructions:

Carefully pour the lye into the distilled water. Stir gently until the lye is dissolved.

Set aside the lye solution and allow to cool.

Mix the first 5 oils together.

Carefully pour the lye and water solution into the oils. Stir all the ingredients together.

Add the activated charcoal.

Using a hand mixer, blend the soap mixture until you get a creamy pudding consistency.

Stir in the lavender essential oil.

Pour the soap mixture into the soap molds. Let the soap to dry for 24 hours before cutting them into bars.

Wrap the soaps in wax paper and store in a cool dry area for curing.

Banish Bacne Soap

Supplies Needed:

2 cups soap base (olive oil)

2 tablespoons bentonite clay

2 tablespoons activated charcoal powder

1 teaspoon tea tree essential oil

1 teaspoon lemongrass essential oil

Soap mold

Instructions:

Cut the olive oil soap base into small cubes and heat in the microwave until completely melted. Make sure to use a heat resistant glass container.

Dissolve the bentonite clay and activated charcoal powder in 1 cup of melted olive oil soap base.

Pour it back into the rest of the olive oil soap base.

Stir in the tea tree and lemongrass essential oils. Mix well before pouring the soap into the molds.

Cut the soap into bars after letting it to dry and harden for 3-4 hours.

Wrap in wax paper and store in a cool place.

Wake Up Fabulous Beauty Soap

Supplies Needed:

2 cups soap base (aloe vera)

2 tablespoons lemongrass essential oil

1 tablespoon clary sage essential oil

Soap mold

Instructions:

Cut aloe vera soap base into small cubes and place in a glass microwaveable bowl.

Heat the soap base in the microwave in 20 second intervals until it's completely melted.

Allow the aloe vera soap base to cool for 5 minutes before stirring in the lemongrass and clary sage essential oils.

Pour the soap mixture into the mold and set aside. Let it harden for 3-4 hours before cutting it into bars.

Wrap soap bars in wax paper and store in a cool dry place.

Minty Fresh Summer Bar

Supplies Needed:

2 cups soap base (cocoa butter)

1 tablespoon loose dried mint leaves

2 tablespoons neroli essential oil

1 tablespoons eucalyptus essential oil

Soap mold

Instructions:

Cut the cocoa butter soap base into small cubes. Place the cubes in a glass bowl.

Heat the soap base in the microwave in 20 second intervals until completely melted.

Allow the soap base to cool for 5 minutes before stirring in the essential oils.

Add half of the dried mint leaves and whisk to mix the ingredients together.

Pour soap into the mold.

Sprinkle the remaining dried mint leaves on top of the soap and set aside for 4-5 hours.

Once the soap is hard, remove from the mold and wrap it in wax paper.

Store in a cool dry place, away from direct sunlight.

Silky Smooth Bath Soap

Supplies Needed:

3 cups soap base (goat's milk)

1 cup goat's milk powder

2 tablespoons sandalwood essential oil

1 tablespoon rose essential oil

1 tablespoon patchouli essential oil

Soap mold

Instructions:

Cut goat's milk soap base into small cubes and place in a heat resistant microwave safe bowl.

Heat soap base in the microwave in 20 second intervals until it's melted.

Allow soap base to cool for 5 minutes before adding the essential oils.

Add goat's milk powder into the soap mixture and whisk until you get a creamy consistency.

Pour the soap mixture into the mold.

Set aside the soap for 4-5 hours to harden.

Cut the soap into bars and wrap it in wax paper. Store it in a cool dry place.

Spots Be Gone Clarifying Bar

Supplies Needed:

2 cups soap base (cocoa butter)

½ cup bentonite clay

¼ cup distilled water

2 tablespoons jojoba oil

2 tablespoons castor oil

2 tablespoon lemon essential oil

1 tablespoon frankincense essential oil

Soap mold

Instructions:

Cut cocoa butter soap base into small chunks and melt in a heat resistant microwave safe glass bowl.

Set the microwave to 20 second intervals and heat the soap until it's fully liquefied.

In a separate bowl, mix distilled water and bentonite clay until you get a paste.

Allow the melted soap base to cool for 5 minutes before adding the clay paste and carrier oils.

Stir in the essential oils.

Whisk the soap mixture until you get a creamy consistency.

Pour the soap mixture into the mold and set it aside.

Let it harden overnight before cutting the soap into bars.

Wrap in wax paper. Keep away from direct sunlight.

Brown Sugar Beauty Bar

Supplies Needed:

1 ½ cup soap base (cocoa butter)

3 tablespoons jojoba oil

3 tablespoons distilled water

½ cup brown sugar

1 teaspoon frankincense essential oil

Soap mold

Instructions:

Cut cocoa butter soap base into small cubes.

Put the soap base cubes in a heat resistant glass container and melt for 2-3 minutes in the microwave.

Once the soap base is completely melted, allow it to cool for 5 minutes.

Stir in the jojoba oil and frankincense essential oil.

Mix the brown sugar with water to make a paste.

Whisk all the ingredients together until the soap mixture thickens.

Pour the coffee soap mixture into the mold.

Leave the soap to harden overnight.

Take the soap out of the mold and cut into bars.

Wrap soap in wax paper and store in a cool place, away from direct sunlight.

Autumn Kiss Nourishing Soap

Supplies Needed:

2 cups soap base (shea butter)

1 cup cornmeal

2 tablespoons almond oil

1 tablespoon clove essential oil

Soap mold

Instructions:

Spread out half of the cornmeal at the bottom of the soap mold.

Cut the shea butter soap base into cubes.

Put shea butter soap cubes in a microwave safe glass container and melt for around 45 seconds in the microwave. Take the soap base out of the microwave, give it a stir, and put it back into the microwave for a minute until it's completely melted.

Allow the soap base to cool for 5 minutes.

Stir in the almond oil and clove essential oil. Add the remaining cornmeal into the soap base and whisk all the ingredients together.

Pour the soap mixture into the mold.

Set aside the soap mixture and allow it to cure for at least 24 hours before taking it out of the mold.

Take the soap out of the mold and cut into bars with a sharp knife.

Store soap in wax paper and keep away from direct sunlight.

Happy Days Soap

Supplies Needed:

3 cups soap base (olive oil)

½ cup dried jasmine flowers

2 tablespoons jasmine essential oil

1 tablespoon lavender essential oil

Soap mold

Instructions:

Cut olive oil soap base into small chunks and put in a microwave safe glass container.

Melt the olive oil soap base in the microwave in 30 second intervals until you get a liquefied soap.

Set aside the liquefied soap and let it to cool for 5 minutes.

While waiting for the soap to cool, crumble the dried jasmine flowers.

Stir in jasmine and lavender essential oils. Add more if you want the scent to be stronger.

Whisk in the dried jasmine flowers.

Pour the soap mixture into a mold. Allow the soap to cure overnight.

Pop the soap out of the mold and wrap it in wax paper.

Store soap in a cool dry place, away from direct heat and sunlight.

Sahara Daydreams Nourishing Bar

Supplies Needed:

3 cups soap base (cocoa butter)

1 tablespoon lemon essential oil

1 tablespoon patchouli essential oil

½ tablespoon ginger essential oil

¼ teaspoon red mica powder

¼ teaspoon blue mica powder

1 tablespoon distilled water

Soap mold

Instructions:

Cut the cocoa butter soap base into small cubes and put in a heat resistant glass microwaveable bowl.

Heat the cocoa butter soap base in the microwave in 30 second intervals until it's fully melted.

Set aside the liquefied cocoa butter soap base and let it to cool for 5 minutes.

Stir in all the essential oils and mix well.

Dissolve the red and blue mica powders in 1 tablespoon of distilled water before adding it to the cocoa butter soap base. Mix well until you get an even purple hue.

Pour the soap mixture into the mold.

Allow the soap to cure for 5-6 hours before popping it out of the mold.

Slice the soap into bars and wrap it in wax paper.

Keep away from direct heat and sunlight.

Safe for Baby Nourishing Bar

Supplies Needed:

3 ounce coconut oil

2 ounce shea butter

1 ounce castor oil

.87 ounce lye

1.98 ounce distilled water

Soap mold

Instructions:

Carefully pour the lye into the distilled water. Stir gently until the lye is dissolved.

Set aside the lye solution and allow to cool.

Mix coconut oil, shea butter, and castor oil together.

Carefully pour the lye and water solution into the oils. Stir all the ingredients together.

Using a hand mixer, blend the soap mixture until you get a creamy pudding consistency.

Pour the soap mixture into the soap molds. Let the soap to dry for 24 hours before cutting them into bars.

Wrap the soaps in wax paper and store in a cool dry area to cure. Recommended curing period 2-4 weeks.

Eczema Buster Smoothening Soap

Supplies Needed:

3 ounce coconut oil

2 ounce extra virgin olive oil

1 ounce jojoba oil

.80 ounce lye

1.98 ounce distilled water

20 drops tea tree essential oil

Soap mold

Instructions:

Carefully pour the lye into the distilled water. Stir gently until the lye is dissolved.

Set aside the lye solution and allow to cool.

Mix the first 3 oils together.

Carefully pour the lye and water solution into the oils. Stir all the ingredients together.

Using a hand mixer, blend the soap mixture until you get a creamy pudding consistency.

Stir in the tea tree essential oil.

Pour the soap mixture into the soap molds. Let the soap to dry for 24 hours before cutting them into bars.

Wrap the soaps in wax paper and store in a cool dry area for curing.

Naturally Fresh Deodorant Soap

Supplies Needed:

2 cups soap base (aloe vera)

2 tablespoons dried calendula flowers

1 tablespoon tea tree essential oil

1 tablespoon peppermint essential oil

½ tablespoon bergamot essential oil

½ tablespoon lemon essential oil

Soap mold

Instructions:

Cut the aloe vera soap base into small cubes and heat in the microwave until completely melted. Make sure to use a heat resistant glass container.

Allow the soap base to cool for 5 minutes before adding the dried calendula flowers.

Stir in the tea tree, peppermint, bergamot, and lemon essential oils. Mix well before pouring the soap mixture into the mold.

Cut the soap into bars after letting it dry for 24 hours.

Wrap individual soap bars in wax paper and store in a cool place.

Citrus Energizing Soap

Supplies Needed:

1 ½ cup soap base (aloe vera)

2 tablespoons dried lemon rind

1 tablespoon sweet orange essential oil

1 tablespoon grapefruit essential oil

Soap mold

Instructions:

Cut aloe vera soap base into small cubes and place in a glass microwaveable bowl.

Heat the soap base in the microwave in 20 second intervals until it's completely melted.

Allow the aloe vera soap base to cool for 5 minutes before stirring in the sweet orange and grapefruit essential oils.

Add the dried lemon rind into the soap base and whisk to combine all the ingredients.

Pour the soap mixture into the mold and set aside. Let it harden for 3-4 hours before cutting it into bars.

Wrap soap bars in wax paper and store in a cool dry place.

Ginger Rose Loofah Soap

Supplies Needed:

2 cups soap base (glycerin)

2 tablespoons rose essential oil

½ teaspoon ginger essential oil

¼ teaspoon yellow mica powder

Loofah

Soap mold

Instructions:

Cut the glycerin soap base into small cubes. Place the cubes in a glass bowl.

Heat the soap base in the microwave in 20 second intervals until completely melted.

Allow the soap base to cool for 5 minutes before stirring in the essential oils.

Add the yellow mica powder to the soap mixture and mix.

Cut the loofah so that it fits snugly into the soap mold.

Pour the soap mixture into the mold.

Set the soap aside for at least 6 hours.

Once the soap is hard, remove from the mold, and cut it into bars.

Store in a cool dry place, away from direct sunlight.

Spiced Soap for Men

Supplies Needed:

4 ounce tallow

2 ounce coconut oil

2 ounce olive oil

1 ounce castor oil

2 ounce beeswax

1.34 ounce lye

3.63 ounce distilled water

20 drops patchouli essential oil

20 drops sweet orange essential oil

10 drops cinnamon essential oil

Soap mold

Instructions:

Carefully pour the lye into the distilled water. Stir gently until the lye is dissolved.

Set aside the lye solution and allow to cool.

Warm the beeswax in a pot on low heat until completely melted. Carefully add the first 5 oils one at a time. Make sure that the oils don't get too hot.

Take the pot off the heat.

Carefully pour the lye and water solution into a pot. Stir all the ingredients together.

Using a hand mixer, blend the soap mixture until you get a creamy pudding consistency.

Put the pot back on low heat and let the soap mixture to cook for about an hour or until the mixture turns transparent.

Stir in the patchouli, sweet orange, and cinnamon essential oils.

Pour the soap mixture into the soap molds. Let the soap to dry for 24 hours before cutting them into bars.

Wrap the soaps in wax paper and store in a cool dry area for curing. Recommended time is around 2-4 weeks.

Sweet Surrender Creamy Shaving Bar

Supplies Needed:

3 cups soap base (goat's milk)

1 tablespoon glycerin

2 tablespoons bentonite clay

1 tablespoon sweet orange essential oil

1 tablespoon lavender essential oil

Soap mold

Instructions:

Cut goat's milk soap base into small cubes and place in a heat resistant microwave safe bowl.

Heat soap base in the microwave in 20 second intervals until it's melted.

Allow soap base to cool for before adding the bentonite clay.

Add the glycerin and essential oils.

Whisk the soap mixture until you get a creamy consistency.

Pour the soap mixture into the mold.

Set aside the soap for at least 6 hours to harden.

Cut the soap into bars and wrap it in wax paper. Store it in a cool dry place.

Mountain Breeze Cleansing Bar

Supplies Needed:

2 cups soap base (glycerin)

½ cup activated charcoal

¼ cup distilled water

2 tablespoons cedar wood essential oil

1 tablespoon lemongrass essential oil

Soap mold

Instructions:

Cut the glycerin soap base into small chunks and melt in a heat resistant microwave safe glass bowl.

Set the microwave to 20 second intervals and heat the soap base until it's fully liquefied.

In a separate bowl, mix the activated charcoal with the distilled water until you get a paste.

Allow the melted soap base to cool for 5 minutes before stirring in the essential oils.

Add the activated charcoal paste to the soap base.

Whisk the soap mixture until you get a thick consistency.

Pour the soap mixture into the mold and set it aside.

Let it harden for at least 6 hours before cutting the soap into bars.

Wrap in wax paper. Keep away from direct sunlight.

Sweet Avocado Soothing Bar

Supplies Needed:

4 ounce avocado oil

3 ounce palm kernel oil

3 ounce palm oil

2 ounce beeswax

1.57 ounce lye

3.96 ounce distilled water

20 drops sweet almond oil

Soap mold

Instructions:

Carefully pour the lye into the distilled water. Stir gently until the lye is dissolved.

Set aside the lye solution and allow to cool.

Warm the beeswax in a pot on low heat until completely melted. Carefully add the first 4 oils one at a time. Make sure that the oils don't get too hot.

Take the pot off the heat.

Carefully pour the lye and water solution into a pot. Stir all the ingredients together.

Using a hand mixer, blend the soap mixture until you get a creamy pudding consistency.

Put the pot back on low heat and let the soap mixture to cook for about an hour or until the mixture turns transparent.

Stir in the sweet almond oil.

Pour the soap mixture into the soap molds. Let the soap to cure for 24 hours before cutting them into bars.

Wrap the soaps in wax paper and store in a cool dry area.

Healing Balm Soap

Supplies Needed:

4 ounce coconut oil

4 ounce olive oil

1 ounce castor oil

2 ounce sunflower oil

2 ounce beeswax

1.7 ounce lye

4.29 ounce distilled water

20 drops lemongrass essential oil

20 drops lime essential oil

Soap mold

Instructions:

Carefully pour the lye into the distilled water. Stir gently until the lye is dissolved.

Set aside the lye solution and allow to cool.

Warm the beeswax in a pot on low heat until completely melted. Carefully add the first 4 oils one at a time. Make sure that the oils don't get too hot.

Take the pot off the heat.

Carefully pour the lye and water solution into the pot. Stir all the ingredients together.

Using a hand mixer, blend the soap mixture until you get a creamy pudding consistency.

Put the pot back on low heat and let the soap mixture to cook for about an hour or until the mixture turns transparent.

Stir in the lemongrass and lime essential oils.

Pour the soap mixture into the soap molds. Let the soap to dry for 24 hours before cutting them into bars.

Wrap the soaps in wax paper and store in a cool dry area for curing.

Mild Chamomile Relaxing Bar

Supplies Needed:

1 ½ cup glycerin soap base (clear)

3 tablespoons olive oil

3 tablespoons chamomile tea

½ cup finely ground oatmeal

1 tablespoon chamomile essential oil

Soap mold

Instructions:

Cut glycerin into small cubes.

Put glycerin cubes in a microwave safe glass container and melt for 2-3 minutes in the microwave.

Once the glycerin is melted, allow it to cool for 5 minutes.

Stir in olive oil and chamomile tea. Add the finely ground oatmeal and chamomile essential oil and whisk it all together.

Mix until the soap mixture begins to thicken.

Pour the chamomile soap mixture into the mold.

Leave the soap mixture to harden overnight.

Take the soap out of the mold and cut into bars.

Wrap soap in wax paper and store in a cool place, away from direct sunlight.

Chapter 12: It's Thyme: Herbal Soap Making From Scratch

Making soaps on your own is not only a great and healthy natural substitute to chemical-based soaps; it is also creative, fulfilling, and thrifty. Plus it's fun, addictive, and could help make you money, too! And that's not even the best part; soap making is pretty easy to do.

Basic Soap Making Methods

Melt and Pour – This is the easiest method. You simply melt store-bought pre-made blocks of all-natural herbal soap and then add your own fragrance.

Cold Process – This is the most common soap-making-from-scratch method, using herbs, oils, and lye.

Hot Process – This is a variation of the cold process but the soap is cooked in a soap pot or an oven.

Rebatching - This involves crushing and grinding herbal soap bars, then adding milk or water, and finally re-blending them.

Cold Process

What you'll need:

A smooth, uncluttered work table with access to running water and a heat source

All the equipment listed in Chapter 4 Animal or vegetable oils of your choice Lye-water based on your recipe Fragrance or essential oil and natural colorant of your choice, optional

The Process

Put on your apron, rubber gloves, and safety goggles and do not remove them until you are completely finished making the soap and all soap making tools have been cleaned and put away.

Get rid of all distractions including pets and small children.

Prepare your equipment. If using wooden molds, line with freezer paper. If using plastic molds, spray with oil based non-stick spray.

Fill the sink or a bowl with ice and some water making an ice bath.

It is imperative to follow the recipe exactly. Weigh all the solid oils. Set aside in a container.

Weigh all the liquid oils. Set aside in another container.

Weigh all the fats. Set aside in a different container.

Weigh all the essential oils. Set aside in a separate container.

Weigh the water or herbal infusion into a heat-proof container.

Heat the fats until completely melted. Remove from heat and then add the liquid oils.

Weigh the lye crystals in a glass jar. Set aside in a safe place.

Weigh the water or herbal infusion again. In its heat-proof container, place the water in the ice bath.

Slowly add all the lye into the water or herbal infusion.

Stick the thermometer in the mix. Stir the lye slowly and carefully until the mixture reduces to around 95°F.

Stir the oil mixture and the lye mix separately using different stirrers. Stir until each mix reaches 80°F. Use warm water baths to regulate the temperatures if needed.

When both reach 80°F, pour the lye into oil slowly and carefully.

Stir gently until well incorporated. Once it is incorporated, you can start using the immersion blender for about 5 to 10 minutes or until you reach the "trace" stage. If mixing by hand, it might take about 15 to 60 minutes. Trace means your soap has emulsified; when the oils and water have mixed well enough and will not separate. To check, dip your spatula or spoon into the mixture and trickle a bit of the mix back into the soap pot. If it leaves a bit of "trace" behind, that's it. The mixture doesn't have to be thick yet, but it needs to be well-mixed enough as to not have streaks of remaining oil.

Once you are on the "trace" stage, add the essential oil, dry herbs, and super fatting oils.

Continue using the blender until the trace thickens.

Pour the mixture into a mold. Cover with

A blanket to insulate and place in a warm area.

Clean your equipment and put them away. Remove your protective clothing.

Set the soap aside for a day.

After 24 hours, remove the blanket and set aside for another day.

After 24 hours, remove the soap from the mold and cut into your desired shape.

Set it aside to cure in open air for 4 to 6 weeks.

Hot Process

What you'll need:

The hot soap making process is very similar to the cold process. They require the tools, the same base ingredients, and combine the ingredients pretty much the same way.

The Process

Put on your apron, rubber gloves, and safety goggles and do not remove them until you are completely finished making the soap and all soap making tools have been cleaned and put away.

Get rid of all distractions including pets and small children. You need a couple of hours for this process.

Measure the ingredients such as natural additives and colorants, and essential oils. Place them in individual containers.

Weigh all the liquid oils. Set aside in another container.

Weigh all the fats. Set aside in a different container.

Weigh all the essential oils. Set aside in a separate container.

Weigh the water or herbal infusion into a heat-proof container.

Weigh the lye crystals in a glass jar. Set aside in a safe place.

In its heat-proof container, place the water in the ice bath.

Slowly add all the lye into the water or herbal infusion. Stir slowly until all the lye crystals are dissolved.

In your soap pot set on low; add the solid oils and stir slowly.

Add in the liquid oils when the solid oils have melted,

Pour a thin stream of the lye-water mix slowly into the oil. Use the whisk or a stick blender to stir.

Keep the stirring motion strong and steady; not too fast but enough to keep the mixture moving. Do this until the lye, water, and oil molecules meet and fuse together to make soap.

Stir thoroughly until the mix becomes thick, creamy and opaque and reach a thick "trace" stage.

Once the soap is in the "trace" stage, put the lid on the pot and leave it on low heat for a several minutes. Watch out for the bubbles around the pot's edges. This may take a while.

The mixture will start looking like a thick gooey Vaseline-like mass. To check if it is done, take a small amount and rub between your fingers. If it feels waxy, then it is done.

Add in dry herbs and fragrance oils if you want.

Quickly scoop the mix into the mold as it tends to harden rapidly.

Set aside for 48 hours. 21.

Remove the soap from the mold and cut into desired size and shape.

Place the soaps on a flat tray lined with paper towels.

Store them in a dry, cool, and dark location for 4 to 6 weeks to cure. The longer you cure, the milder the soap will be.

Chapter 13: Soap Recipes

In this chapter, it will be about recipes, and recipes and more recipes. Since in the previous chapter I have shown you how to make soap, use these ingredients to make your batch.

RECIPE 1:

Veggies Suds 1

0.75 pounds of lye crystals

1 pound of Palm oil

25 ounces of cold water

1.5 pounds of coconut oil

1.5 pounds of olive oil

1.25 pounds of Canola oil or soybean or a mix of both (what's your choice?)

The temperature should be about 230 Fahrenheit and the soap will be hard with a silky lather.

RECIPE 2:

Veggie Suds With Coconut

2.5 pounds of olive oil

1.5 pounds of soybean oil

0.625 pounds of palm oil

26 ounces of cold water

0.875 pounds of coconut oil

0.75 pounds of lye crystals

The temperature of all these ingredients should be 110°C.

RECIPE 3:

Veggies Suds 3

2.5 pounds of olive oil

1.125 pounds of palm oil

1.5 - 1.75 pounds of cold water

1.5 pounds of coconut oil

0.75 pounds of lye crystals

Temperature maintained at 230 Fahrenheit.

RECIPE 4:

Chocolate Almond Soap

O.75 pounds of lye crystals

2 pounds of cold water

1 pound of palm oil

0.875 pounds of coconut oil

0.375 pounds of cocoa butter

3.25 pounds of olive oil

When trace occurs, add:

1 ounce of bitter almond fragrance oil

Blend 2-3 teaspoons of cocoa powder into 1/4 of the soap you are using. The 3/4 of the mixture is already poured into a mold.

The temperature should be at 35^0 to $37.78^{\circ}C$.

Instructions

Add bitter almond oil when you notice trace early enough and pour the rest of the mix into your molds.

Mix cocoa powder immediately to the remaining soap using a stick blender

Drizzle at the top in a back and forth motion.

Using a butter knife, run it back and forth to swirl together the colors.

Blend your powder using some of your soap before mixing it all with the rest of the soap.

RECIPE 5:

Luxury Castile Bar Soap

0.375 pounds of palm oil

1.5 pounds of cold water

0.375 pounds of coconut oil

0.75 pounds of lye crystals

4.875 pounds of olive oil

1.All oils should be heated up to 60°C and the lye solution at 43.33°C.

2.This is a favorite vegetable soap for some soap-makers out there. The result will be a hard and smooth soap with it's supposed to be non-sticky and has no oil seepage.

3.When making this bar of soap and you use a stick blender, trace will set up pretty fast, therefore, it is recommended that you pour the lye at the beginning of the trace. Hard bar of soap will be produced and it will be mild.

4.This soap is great for babies and people who have sensitive skin.

RECIPE 6:

Conclusion

Thank you again for downloading this book!

I hope this book was able to help you to learn how to make soaps.

The next step is to begin adding in all kinds of fragrances and oils to make the soaps all your own.

Thank you and good luck!